For therapists who want an introduction to the history of assessment processes and a thorough presentation of an operative family assessment model, they can find no better one than Family Life Space Drawing by Beeton and Clark. This experienced couple offer a process that is comprehensive and effective for all therapists working with couples and families who want to update their assessment skills.

Harville Hendrix, PhD and **Helen LaKelly Hunt, PhD**, authors of
Getting the Love You Want: A Guide for Couples

Beeton and Clark have made a remarkable contribution to pioneering family therapy assessment resources. Their publication is dedicated to the Family Life Space Drawing, a graphic multilevel assessment instrument. It effectively assists in identifying and utilizing reciprocal and complex communication feedback loops. The authors provide an easy-to-read review of the measure's origins which is backed by theoretical constructs and research. This user-friendly manual includes individual, couples, and family multicultural and international examples taken from a variety of settings. The spatial, symbolic, and social dimensions of the FLSD will provide clinicians and their clients with diversity sensitive clues to their families' sense of emotive closeness and expression. This is an excellent resource for family therapy educators, researchers, and clinicians alike.

Noah Hass-Cohen, PsyD, MA, ATR-BC, Associate Professor, Couples Family Therapy Masters and Doctoral Programs, California School of Professional Psychology

Assessing Family Relationships

Assessing Family Relationships shows mental health professionals how to utilize the Family Life Space Drawing (the FLSD), a family assessment tool that incorporates information from multiple family members while building connections between the clinician and the client.

In this manual, Theresa A. Beeton and Ronald A. Clark demonstrate the usefulness of the FLSD in both family and couple counseling. As a task-centered assessment tool, the FLSD enables an interactive and personalized process of counseling, which helps individuals to express concerns and information about themselves in an indirect and nonthreatening manner. Chapters are illustrated throughout with case studies and drawings adapted from the authors' own clinical experience, and the manual offers an overview of the history of the FLSD and where future research is headed.

Providing a practical explanation of how to complete the FLSD process, *Assessing Family Relationships* will be highly relevant to couple and family therapists, as well as clinical social workers, who are interested in updating their practice with innovative family assessment research and techniques.

Theresa A. Beeton, PhD, LCSW practices as a social worker with a wide range of counseling experience. Currently she is in private practice working with couples and families. Her past professional experiences include work with adoptions, foster care, crisis intervention, as well as many mental health concerns. Additionally, she has taught social workers and mental health students in three different University settings.

Ronald A. Clark, MSW, LCSW is a private practitioner in the area of couple counseling and family therapy. In addition to providing direct services to clients of all ages and backgrounds, he has been a faculty member of the Catholic University of America, teaching graduate students of social work. He came to the mental health field after serving as a Marine Corps officer.

Assessing Family Relationships

A Family Life Space Drawing Manual

Theresa A. Beeton and
Ronald A. Clark

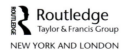
NEW YORK AND LONDON

First published 2019
by Routledge
52 Vanderbilt Avenue, New York, NY 10017

and by Routledge
2 Park Square, Milton Park, Abingdon, Oxon, OX14 4RN

Routledge is an imprint of the Taylor & Francis Group, an informa business

© 2019 Theresa A. Beeton and Ronald A. Clark

The right of Theresa A. Beeton and Ronald A. Clark to be identified as authors of this work has been asserted by them in accordance with sections 77 and 78 of the Copyright, Designs and Patents Act 1988.

All rights reserved. No part of this book may be reprinted or reproduced or utilised in any form or by any electronic, mechanical, or other means, now known or hereafter invented, including photocopying and recording, or in any information storage or retrieval system, without permission in writing from the publishers.

Trademark notice: Product or corporate names may be trademarks or registered trademarks, and are used only for identification and explanation without intent to infringe.

Library of Congress Cataloging-in-Publication Data
A catalog record for this title has been requested

ISBN: 978-1-138-54304-1 (hbk)
ISBN: 978-1-138-54305-8 (pbk)
ISBN: 978-1-351-00752-8 (ebk)

Typeset in Joanna MT & Frutiger
by Apex CoVantage, LLC

https://www.routledge.com/9781138543058

Contents

List of Figures — xvi
List of Tables — xix

PART ONE
Background of Family Assessment and Step-by-Step Instructions for Family Life Space Drawing (FLSD) — 1
Introduction — 1

1 Introducing Methods of Family Assessment — 3
Family Assessment — 3
The Genogram Process — 4
The Strategic Approach — 5
The Structural Approach — 6
The Experiential Model — 7
Psychodynamic Family Therapy — 8
Cognitive Behavioral Family Therapy — 10
Solution-Focused Family Therapy — 11
Narrative Family Therapy — 12
Common Components of Family Assessment — 13
Purpose and Value of Family Assessment — 14
Crucial Qualities of Effective Assessment — 15
The Family Life Space Drawing — 15
Summary — 17
References — 17

2 The Family Life Space Drawing: History and Development of the Process — 20
Danuta Mostwin — 20
Short-Term Multidimensional Family Intervention — 22
Beyond the STMFI Model — 27
Summary — 27
References — 28

3	**Family Life Space Drawing: Theories Behind the Family Life Space Process**	**29**
	Introduction	29
	Systems Theory	30
	Field Theory	31
	Communication Theory	34
	Expressive Therapy Techniques	35
	Other Theoretical Influences	36
	Symbolic Interactionism	36
	Summary	37
	References	37
4	**Family Life Space Drawing: Ten Steps to Complete the Family Life Space Drawing**	**39**
	Symbolic Representation	39
	Ten Steps to Complete the FLSD Process	39
	Step One: Introducing the Process	40
	Step Two: The Facilitator Draws the First Symbol	40
	Step Three: Family Members Each Draw a Personal Symbol	40
	Step Four: Placement of Significant People	41
	Step Five: Environmental or Institutional Factors	42
	Step Six: Identifying Stress Factors	44
	Step Seven: Optional Symbols – Number One Concern, Greatest Frustration	44
	Step Eight: Communication Lines	44
	Step Nine: Reflecting With the Family	45
	Step Ten: Developing the Treatment Plan	46
	FLSD Symbols	46
	Large Symbol	46
	Small Symbol	47
	Environmental or Institutional Symbol	47
	Stress Symbol	47
	Number One Concern Symbol	48
	Greatest Frustration Symbol	48
	Communication Lines Symbol	48
	Symbolic Representation of the FLSD	49
	Summary	49
	References	50
5	**Interpreting the Symbolic Representations of the Family Life Space Drawing**	**51**
	Interpreting the Symbolic Representations of the FLSD	51
	Control Circle	51
	Inner Zone	52
	Middle Zone	53
	Outer Zone	53

CONTENTS | ix

Other Placements	53
Placement of Symbols	54
Distances and Closeness	55
Size of Symbol	55
Interpreting Number One Concern and Greatest Frustration Symbols	55
Obtaining Client Information With the FLSD	56
Ideal Family Representations	57
Ideal Placements	58
Representing Ideal Family Placements: Case Example 5.A	58
Case Example 5.B With Symbolic Interpretation	59
Step Three: Placement of Self	60
Step Four: Placement of Significant Others	61
Key to Symbols	61
Reflections on Wife's Placements	62
Reflections on Husband's Placements	63
Step Five: Environmental Symbols	63
Key to Symbols	63
Reflections on Wife's Environmental Symbols	65
Reflections on Husband's Environmental Symbols	65
Step Six: Stress Symbols	66
Key to Symbols	66
Reflections on Wife's Stress Symbols	67
Reflections on Husband's Stress Symbols	67
Step Seven: Number One Concern and Greatest Frustration Symbols	68
Wife's Placement for Symbol of Number One Concern and Greatest Frustration	68
Husband's Placement for Symbol of Number One Concern and Greatest Frustration	68
Possible Uses of This Information With Case Example 5.B	68
Summary	70
References	70

PART TWO
Using the Family Life Space Drawing (FLSD) With Different Types of Clients

	71
Introduction	71

6	**The Individual Family Life Space Drawing**	**73**
	The Individual FLSD	73
	Individual FLSD: Case Example 6.A	73
	Steps Three and Four: Placement of Self and Significant Others	74
	Placement of Self	74
	Significant Others	75
	Size	75
	Reflections on Steps Three and Four: Individual Case Example 6.A	76

Step Five: Environmental Symbols	76
Key to Symbols	77
Placement	77
Size	77
Distance	77
Reflections on Step Five: Individual Case Example 6.A	77
Step Six: Stress Symbols	77
Placement	78
Size	78
Distance	78
Reflections on Step Six: Individual Case Example 6.A	79
Using the FLSD With Individual Case Example 6.A	79
Individual FLSD: Case Example 6.B	79
Steps Three and Four: Placement of Self, Significant Others	80
Key to Symbols	80
Placement of Self	80
Significant Others	80
Size	80
Distance	80
Reflections on Steps Three and Four: Individual Case Example 6.B	82
Step Five: Environmental Symbols	82
Key to Symbols	82
Placement	82
Size	82
Distance	82
Reflections on Step Five: Individual Case Example 6.B	83
Step Six: Stress Symbols	84
Key to Symbols	84
Placement	85
Size	85
Distance	85
Reflections on Step Six: Individual Case Example 6.B	85
Step Eight: Communication Lines: Individual Case Example 6.B	85
Using the FLSD With Individual Case Example 6.B	86
Individual FLSD: Case Example 6.C	86
Steps Three and Four: Placement of Self and Significant Others	86
Key to Symbols	86
Placement of Self	88
Significant Others	88
Size	88
Distance	88
Reflections on Steps Three and Four: Individual Case Example 6.C	89
Step Five: Environmental Symbols	89
Key to Symbols	89
Placement	89

	Size	89
	Distance	89
	Reflections on Step Five: Individual Case Example 6.C	91
	Step Six: Stress Symbols	91
	Key to Symbols	91
	Placement	92
	Size	92
	Distance	92
	Reflections on Step Six: Individual Case Example 6.C	92
	Step Eight: Communication Lines	93
	Key to Symbols	93
	Reflections on Step Eight: Individual Case Example 6.C	93
	Using the FLSD With Individual Case Example 6.C	93
	Summary: Individual Family Life Space Drawing	93
	References	94
7	**Family Life Space Drawing: Examples With Couples**	**95**
	FLSD With Couples	95
	Couple Case Example 7.A	95
	Step Three: Placement of Self	96
	Reflections on Step Three: Couple Case Example 7.A	96
	Step Four: Placing Significant Others	96
	Key to Symbols	98
	Reflections on Step Four: Couple Case Example 7.A	99
	Step Five: Environmental Symbols	100
	Key to Symbols	100
	Reflections on Step Five: Couple Case Example 7.A	100
	Step Six: Stress Symbols, Example 7.A	101
	Key to Symbols	101
	Reflections on Step Six: Couple Case Example 7.A	101
	Step Eight: Communication Lines	103
	Key to Symbols	103
	Reflections on Step Eight: Couple Case Example 7.A	103
	Using the FLSD With Couple Case Example 7.A	103
	Couple Case Example 7.B	104
	Step Three: Placement of Self	104
	Step Four: Placement of Significant Others	106
	Key to Symbols (Wife)	106
	Key to Symbols (Husband)	106
	Reflections on Step Four: Couple Case Example 7.B	106
	Step Five: Environmental Symbols	108
	Key to Symbols (Husband)	108
	Key to Symbols (Wife)	108
	Placement	110
	Distance	110

Reflections on Step Five: Couples Case Example 7.B		111
Step Six: Stress Symbols		111
Key to Symbols		111
Reflections on Step Six (Husband): Couple Case Example 7.B		111
Placement		111
Size		111
Distance		113
Reflections on Step Six (Wife): Couple Case Example 7.B		113
Placement		113
Size		113
Distance		113
Reflections		113
Step Seven: Number One Concern and Greatest Frustration (Not Illustrated)		113
Using This Drawing With This Couple Case Example 7.B		113
Couple Case Example 7.C		114
Step Three: Placement of Self		114
Key to Symbols		115
Reflections on Step Three: Couple Case Example 7.C		116
Step Four: Placement of Significant Others		116
Key to Symbols		117
Reflections on Step Four (Female Placements): Couple Case Example 7.C		118
Reflections on Step Four (Male Placements): Couple Case Example 7.C		119
Step Five: Environmental Symbols		119
Key to Symbols		120
Reflections on Step Five (Female): Couple Case Example 7.C		121
Reflections on Step Five (Male): Couple Case Example 7.C		121
Step Six: Stress Symbols		121
Key to Symbols		122
Reflections on Step Six (Female): Couple Case Example 7.C		122
Reflections on Step Six (Male): Couple Case Example 7.C		123
Using the FLSD With Couple Case Example 7.C		124
Summary of Using FLSD With Couples		124
8	**Family Life Space Drawing With Families**	**125**
Families and the FLSD		125
Blended Family: Case Example 8.A		125
Step Three: Placement of Self		126
Key to Symbols		126
Reflections on Step Three: Family Case Example 8.A		126
Step Four: Placement of Significant Others		128
Key to Symbols		128
Reflections on Step Four: Family Case Example 8.A		128
Step Five: Environmental Symbols		131
Key to Symbols		131
Reflections on Step Five: Family Case Example 8.A		133
Step Six: Stress Symbols		134

Key to Symbols		134
Reflections on Step Six: Family Case Example 8.A		134
Step Eight: Communication Lines		137
Reflections on Step Eight: Family Case Example 8.A		139
Using the FLSD With Family Case Example 8.A		140
Family Case Example 8.B		140
Step Three: Placement of Symbols of Self		141
Key to Symbols		141
Reflections on Step Three: Family Case Example 8.B		142
Step Four: Significant Others		142
Key to Symbols		143
Reflections on Step Four: Family Case Example 8.B		144
Step Five: Environmental Symbols		145
Key to Symbols		146
Reflections on Step Five: Family Case Example 8.B		147
Step Six: Stress Symbols		148
Key to Symbols		149
Reflections on Step Six: Family Case Example 8.B		150
Using the FLSD With Family Case Example 8.B		151
Summary: FLSD With Families		151
References		152
9	**Family Life Space Drawing (FLSD) in Various Counseling Settings**	**153**
	FLSD in Various Counseling Settings	153
	Social Service Settings	154
	Foster Care and Adoption	154
	Supporting People in Poverty	155
	Immigrants	156
	Aging Services	156
	Foster Care and Termination of Parental Rights: Case Example 9.A	157
	Step Three: Placement of Self	158
	Step Four: Placement of Significant Others	159
	Key to Symbols	159
	Reflections on Step Four: Case Example 9.A	160
	Step Five: Environmental Symbols (Not Illustrated)	161
	Step Six: Stress Symbols (Not Illustrated)	161
	Using the FLSD With Case Example 9.A	161
	Psychiatric Settings	162
	Psychiatric Facility: Case Example 9.B	163
	Step Three: Placement of Self	163
	Key to Symbols	163
	Step Four: Placement of Significant Others	164
	Step Four: Distance of Symbols	165
	Steps Five and Six: Environmental and Stress Symbols	165
	Step Eight: Communication Lines	165
	School Settings	167

	School Settings: Case Example 9.C	167
	Step Three: Placement of Family Members	168
	Step Four: Placement of Significant Others (Not Illustrated)	168
	Step Five: Environmental Factors (Not Illustrated)	168
	Step Six: Stress Symbols (Not Illustrated)	169
	Step Eight: Communication Lines (Not Illustrated)	169
	Using the FLSD With Case Example 9.C	170
	Treating the Mental Health Needs of Deaf Culture	171
	Summary: The FLSD in Human Services Settings	171
	References	172
10	**Family Life Space Drawing and Research: Past, Present, and Future**	**174**
	Research and the FLSD	174
	Early Research of Short-Term Multidimensional Family Intervention (STMFI) and the Family Life Space Drawing (FLSD)	174
	The FLSD as a Research Device	176
	Other Uses of the FLSD in Research	179
	Researching Expressive Graphic Techniques	179
	Future Research	180
	FLSD Pilot Studies	180
	Pilot Study One: Family Assessment Measure (FAM-III) and the FLSD	181
	FAM-III and the FLSD: Couple Case Example 10.A	181
	Steps Three and Four: Placement of Self and Significant Others	181
	Key to Symbols	181
	FAM-III Scores: Couple Case Example 10.A	182
	FAM-III and the FLSD: Couple Case Example 10.B	184
	Steps Three and Four: Placement of Self and Significant Others	184
	Key to Symbols	184
	FAM-III Scores: Couple Case Example 10.B	185
	FAM-III and the FLSD: Couple Case Example 10.C	186
	Steps Three and Four: Placement of Self and Significant Others	186
	Key to Symbols	186
	FAM-III Scores: Couple Case Example 10.C	188
	Summary of FAM-III Results and the FLSD	188
	Pilot Study Two: FLSD Compared to Experiences in Close Relationship Survey (ECR-R)	188
	FLSD and the ECR-R: Couple Case Example 10.D	189
	Steps Three and Four: Placement of Self and Significant Others	189
	Key to Symbols	189
	ECR-R Scores, Anxiety and Avoidance: Couple Case Example 10.D	189
	FLSD and ECR-R Comparisons: Couple Case Example 10.D	191
	FLSD and ECR-R: Case Example 10.E	191
	Steps Three and Four: Placement of Self and Significant Others	191
	Key to Symbols	191
	ECR-R Results: Couple Case Example 10.E	193

FLSD and ECR-R Comparisons: Couple Case Example 10.E ... 193
FLSD and ECR-R: Couple Case Example 10.F ... 194
    Steps Three and Four: Placement of Self and Significant Others ... 194
    Key to Symbols ... 194
ECR-R Scores: Case Example 10.F ... 195
FLSD and ECR-R Comparisons: Case Example 10.F ... 196
Summary of Pilot Studies ... 196
Future Research ... 196
Summary ... 197
References ... 198

Index ... 200

Figures

1.1	Example of genogram with three-generation family	5
1.2	Example of lines used in Minuchin's family mapping process	6
1.3	Example of family mapping	7
1.4	Example of an ecomap diagram with connection lines	9
1.5	Solution-focused therapy progress scale	11
1.6	Example of narrative problem mapping process	12
3.1	This picture illustrates that the circle with a p in the middle stands for person affected by driving forces on two sides working toward a goal that is obstructed by a barrier	32
4.1	Large family symbol	46
4.2	Self and significant other symbols	47
4.3	Environmental symbols	47
4.4	Stress symbols	47
4.5	Number one concern	48
4.6	Greatest frustration	48
4.7	Good communication line	48
4.8	So-so communication line	48
4.9	Poor communication line	49
5.1	Control circle, zones, and regions	52
5.2	Example of ideal placements in FLSD	58
5.3	Step three: placement of self, Example 5.B	60
5.4	Step four: placement of significant others, Example 5.B	61
5.5	Step five: environmental symbols, Example 5.B	64
5.6	Step six: stress symbols, Example 5.B	66
5.7	Step seven: greatest concern and frustration, Example 5.B	69

FIGURES

6.1	Steps three and four: placement of self and significant others, Example 6.A	74
6.2	Step five: environmental symbols, Example 6.A	76
6.3	Step six: stress symbols, Example 6.A	78
6.4	Steps three and four: placement of self and significant others, Example 6.B	81
6.5	Step five: environmental symbols, Example 6.B	83
6.6	Step six: stress symbols, Example 6.B	84
6.7	Steps three and four: placement of self and significant others, Example 6.C	87
6.8	Step five: environmental symbols, Example 6.C	90
6.9	Steps six and eight: stress symbols and communication lines, Example 6.C	91
7.1	Step three, placing individual symbol: couple case, Example 7.A	97
7.2	Step four, placement of significant others: couple case, Example 7.A	98
7.3	Step five, environmental symbols: couple case, Example 7.A	101
7.4	Step six, stress symbols: couple case, Example 7.A	102
7.5	Step three, placement of self: couple case, Example 7.B	105
7.6	Step four, placement of significant others: couple case, Example 7.B	107
7.7	Step five, environmental symbols: couple case, Example 7.B	109
7.8	Step six, stress symbols: couple case, Example 7.B	112
7.9	Step three, placing individual symbol: couple case, Example 7.C	115
7.10	Step four, placing significant others: couple case, Example 7.C	116
7.11	Step five, environmental symbols: couple case, Example 7.C	120
7.12	Step six, stress symbols: couple case, Example 7.C	122
8.1	Step three, placement of self: family case, Example 8.A	127
8.2	Step four, drawing significant others: family case, Example 8.A	130
8.3	Step five, environmental symbols: family case, Example 8.A	132
8.4	Step six, stress symbols: family case, Example 8.A	135
8.5	Step three, family members place their own symbols: family case, Example 8.B	141
8.6	Step four, placement of significant others: family case, Example 8.B	143
8.7	Step five, environmental symbols: family case, Example 8.B	146
8.8	Step six, stress symbols: family case, Example 8.B	149
9.1	Step three, placement of self: family case, Example 9.A	158
9.2	Step four, placement of significant others: family case, Example 9.A	159
9.3	Steps three and four: placement of self and significant others, Example 9.B	163

9.4	Step three, placement of family members: family case, Example 9.C	169
10.1	Steps three and four: placement of self and significant others, Example 10.A	183
10.2	Steps three and four: placement of self and significant others, Example 10.B	185
10.3	Steps three and four: placement of self and significant others, Example 10.C	187
10.4	Steps three and four: placement of self and significant others, Example 10.D	190
10.5	Steps three and four: placement of self and significant others, Example 10.E	192
10.6	Steps three and four: placement of self and significant others, couple case, Example 10.F	194

Tables

5.1	Placement zone, region, size, and distance, Example 5.A	60
5.2	Significant others: zone and region, Example 5.B	62
5.3	Significant others: size and distance, Example 5.B	62
5.4	Environmental symbols: zones, region, size, and distance, Example 5.B	64
5.5	Step six, stress symbols: zone, region, size, and distance, Example 5.B	67
5.6	Step seven, optional symbols: number one concern (?) and greatest frustration (X), Example 5.B	68
6.1	Steps three and four: zone, region placement, and size, Example 6.A	75
6.2	Step four, significant others: distance from symbol for self, Example 6.A	75
6.3	Step five, environmental symbols: zone, region, size, and distance, Example 6.A	77
6.4	Steps three and four, placement of self and significant others: zone, region, size, and distance, Example 6.B	81
6.5	Step five: environmental symbols, Example 6.B	83
6.6	Step six, stress symbols: zone, region, size, and distance, Example 6.B	84
6.7	Steps three and four: zone, region, size, and distance, Example 6.C	87
6.8	Step three, significant others: distance, Example 6.C	88
6.9	Step five, environmental symbols: zone, region, size, and distance, Example 6.C	90
6.10	Step six, stress symbols: zone, region, size, and distance, Example 6.C	92
7.1	Step three: placement of self, Example 7.A	97
7.2	Step four, significant others: region and zone placements, Example 7.A	99
7.3	Step four, significant others: size and distance, Example 7.A	99
7.4	Step five, environmental symbols: zone, region, size, and distance, Example 7.A	100
7.5	Step six, stress symbols: zone, region, size, and distance, Example 7.A	102
7.6	Step three: zone, region, placement, size, and distance, Example 7.B	105

7.7	Step four, significant others: zone, region, placement, size, and distance, Example 7.B	107
7.8	Step five, environmental symbols: zones, regions, size, and distance, Example 7.B	109
7.9	Step five: distances, husband, Example 7.B	110
7.10	Step five: distances, wife, Example 7.B	110
7.11	Step six, stress symbols: zone, region, size, and distance, Example 7.B	112
7.12	Step three: placement of symbol for self, Example 7.C	115
7.13	Step four, significant others: zone, region, size, and distance, Example 7.C	117
7.14	Step five, environmental symbols: zone, region, size, and distance, Example 7.C	120
7.15	Step six, stress symbols: zone, region, size, and distance, Example 7.C	123
8.1	Step three, placement of self: zone, region, and size, Example 8.A	127
8.2	Step four, significant others: zone placements, Example 8.A	129
8.3	Step four, significant other: size and distance, Example 8.A	130
8.4	Step five, environmental symbols: placements, regions, and zones, Example 8.A	132
8.5	Step five, environmental symbols: size and distance, Example 8.A	133
8.6	Step six: stress symbols, Example 8.A	135
8.7	Step six, size and distance, Example 8.A	136
8.8	Step three: placement of symbols for family members, Example 8.B	142
8.9	Step four, significant others: zone and region, Example 8.B	144
8.10	Step four: size and distance, Example 8.B	144
8.11	Step five, environmental symbols: zones and regions, Example 8.B	147
8.12	Step five, environmental symbols: size and distance, Example 8.B	147
8.13	Step six, stress symbols: zone and region, Example 8.B	150
8.14	Step six, stress symbols: size and distance, Example 8.B	150
9.1	Step three: placements of self, Example 9.A	158
9.2	Step four, placement of others: zone and region, Example 9.A	160
9.3	Step three, placement of self: zone, region, and size, Example 9.B	164
9.4	Step four, significant others: zone and region, Example 9.B	164
9.5	Step three: zone, region, distance, and size, Example 9.C	168
10.1	Step three and four, placement of self, significant others: region, zone, size, and distance, Example 10.A	182

10.2	FAM-III scores, Example 10.A	183
10.3	Steps three and four, placement of self, significant others: region, zone, size, and distance, Example 10.B	184
10.4	FAM-III scores, Example 10.B	186
10.5	Steps three and four, placement of self, significant others: region, zone, size, and distance, Example 10.C	187
10.6	FAM-III scores, Example 10.C	188
10.7	Steps three and four, placement of self, significant others: zone, size, region, and distance, Example 10.D	190
10.8	ECR-R scores for anxiety and avoidance, Example 10.D	191
10.9	Steps three and four, placement of self, significant others: zone, region, size, and distance, Example 10.E	192
10.10	ECR-R subscale scores, Example 10.E	193
10.11	Steps three and four, placement of self, significant others: zone, size, and distance, Example 10.F	195
10.12	ECR-R scores, Example 10.F	196

PART ONE
Background of Family Assessment and Step-by-Step Instructions for Family Life Space Drawing (FLSD)

INTRODUCTION

This manual has been written for the purpose of providing a detailed guide to mental health therapists and other professionals who are interested in a unique information gathering process when working with clients. The Family Life Space Drawing (FLSD) is an assessment and diagnostic process that engages the client in an exercise that allows the client to symbolically inform the therapist and other participants about themselves, their environmental factors, and the stresses having impact on them and others in their life. The authors have been using the FLSD since the 1970s with all types of clients, individuals, couples, and families. Throughout the years both authors have used it in their own clinical practice and presented the FLSD at various national and international conferences, mental health and social service agencies, and a range of institutions of higher learning. Developing the FLSD creates a very positive beginning session when connecting with the client. Even very reluctant clients are usually willing participants with very little urging. When the client is asked to symbolically draw himself or herself on a chart, they place themselves in a position that they see themselves in the family. They will follow through and place other significant persons and other symbols on the chart. It is amazing how responsive they are to following the directions of the therapist.

We want to share this fascinating assessment tool with others because of our experience and expertise in using it for decades, and we know that our mental health colleagues would find it useful in working with clients in their professional settings. We have found it to be an excellent joining instrument for connecting with clients at a deep level. What makes this assessment instrument so special and unique is its simplicity and ease of use. The client provides intimate details about their life with little urging. Using symbols to represent such details frees the client up and they are able to express details about themselves and others without hesitation. Not only is the FLSD an incredible vehicle for information gathering and assessment, the treatment process begins at the onset of the first session. Interacting with the therapist symbolically in the first session helps the client learn how to better express themselves and improve their communication skills when interacting with others.

When clients have completed the FLSD, they are able to observe and reflect on the completed drawing. Usually they respond with insight and often surprise on what is represented so graphically on the FLSD. The client is able to see how each component represented in the FLSD is affected by other components regardless of whether it is another individual, an environmental factor or a stressful event impacting on them or others identified on the drawing. We are excited to share this information and know that it will have value to the mental health and human service community and all the people they serve.

We have divided this manual into two parts. The first part of the manual covers information related to the concept of family assessment in general and reviews the ways that different models of family therapy might assess family situations for treatment. The history of the early creation and usages of the FLSD also give an idea on the early usages of the FLSD process. Part One also reviews the theories that supported the development of the interactive symbolic process. The final chapters of Part One of this manual inform the reader on the specific steps necessary to conduct the FLSD and also provide some information on potential ways to understand the symbolic placements.

Part Two of the manual demonstrates case example of using the FLSD with different types of clients and populations. Chapters focus on specific examples of using the FLSD with individuals, couples, and families. Chapter 9 illustrates the broad use of the FLSD by sharing specific examples of how the FLSD has been used in various human service settings. The final chapter discusses research related to the FLSD and discusses some of the potential possibilities for future research connected to the FLSD constructs.

CHAPTER ONE
Introducing Methods of Family Assessment

FAMILY ASSESSMENT

Sitting in the waiting room of the counseling office is a family looking for help and support regarding a family crisis related to one of their children. The family has never been to a counseling center before and feels a little nervous about having to go outside their inner circle in order to tackle this situation. The child's guidance counselor at the school suggested that the family try some counseling as a way to attend to behavior and management issues with the child. The parents want to be good parents and they feel overwhelmed and out of answers, so they are ready to use whatever resources that might be available to help them with their child. Still, the family is somewhat uncertain as to what will happen once they enter that counseling session. They have seen some counseling sessions on television and movies and wonder if the counseling session will have any resemblance to what they have seen portrayed in the media.

On the other side of the waiting room door is a counselor, possibly trained as a social worker, psychologist, marriage and family therapist, or some other licensed professional counselor. The first session for the client can take many forms and variations, all depending on the type of training and clinical background of the counselor. This same family in the waiting room could have a very different first session experience depending on the training and therapeutic orientations that the counselor decides to take.

Some family counselors will want to have identifying information about the client and family members and will want to know information regarding ages and backgrounds of everyone in the family, even before the session starts. The counselor might ask the clients to fill out lengthy forms online or in the waiting room. Some therapists will want to know about the family in terms of its history and learn about recent and past events that influence the current family situation, while other counselors will just want to talk about the immediate situation of the clients without exploring history. The kinds of information shared in the first session will be directed by the counselor's theoretical orientation, which influences the whole focus of the first session.

Most family therapists operate from a systemic orientation, and family counseling can take on many varieties of applications. Systems theory as it applies to family counseling (discussed in more detail in later chapters) understands problems in a way that explores all aspects of the family or "system" and addresses broader examinations of individual mental health experiences (Fogarty, 1976). Family counselors who want to approach the problem from a systemic perspective will explore the presenting issue from the perspective of the whole group and not just the vantage point of the individual. Understanding the whole family can be assessed by investigating the individual and asking about the family, or it can be assessed by interviewing the whole family at the same time all together. Both perspectives can be identified as family assessment if the whole picture of the person is addressed.

There are many approaches to working with families and many theoretical orientations to addressing counseling situations. Nichols and Davis (2017, p. 258) identifies several models of family therapy, such as Bowenian, strategic, structural, experiential, psychodynamic, cognitive behavioral, solution-focused, and narrative. Each of these models has specific constructs and techniques related to their approach to therapy. The various approaches will take on different paths to assessment and first family sessions. There may be one mountain to climb but many ways and directions to achieve the summit.

Bowenian therapy is concerned with family of origin concerns and focuses on family history. Goals of this type of therapy helps clients to differentiate from family stress, anxieties, and dysfunctional interactions. Clients are encouraged to create new communication patterns that avoid triangular relationships, which are considered inherently dysfunctional (Bowen, 1978). Bowenian family therapy uses a structured assessment and therapeutic process that explores family history and the relationship of individuals within the family. Kerr and Bowen (1988) indicate that family evaluation will explore the history of the presenting problem, the history of the nuclear family, and the history of the extended family system. Often the information obtained from the family is illustrated in visual form by a family diagram (Kerr & Bowen, 1998, p. 306). The family diagram portrays family structure and usually depicts three generations. This process is more commonly identified as a genogram. The genogram maps out the people in the family and looks for generational relationships and problems (McGoldrick, Gerson, & Petry, 2008, p. 5). The genogram can illustrate family patterns in terms of marriages, births, and deaths. Many counselors use the visual to show relationship cutoffs and close connections

The Genogram Process

The genogram process is widely used by counselors. While credit for developing and utilizing the process is given to Murray Bowen and his theories of family systems therapy, this process is used by therapists who follow other theories and orientations of family therapy (McGoldrick et al., 2008, p. 237). Therapists can use this process to engage families, reframe and detoxify family issues, unblock systems, clarify patterns, connect families to their histories, and provide psychoeducational information to clients (McGoldrick et al., 2008).

Bowen's family systems theory uses the information from the family diagram or genogram as a way to visually and symbolically present family history that includes emotional references and connections to people and events in the history. Bowen's family therapy is designed to help people decrease anxiety and form a healthy differentiation of self. Bowenian therapists will look for patterns of emotional cutoff and for information related to lack of differentiation between family members. The genogram visual can help the therapist identify the patterns that prevent healthy differentiation. The visual also directs the conversation toward discovery of new insights and adoption of new behaviors in the family.

The process of completing a genogram or family diagram can take on different directions and meanings depending on the way in which the counselor wants to use and direct the information. In its simplest form, the genogram is a simple and pictorial way to collect information about the client and learn about family history. In a more complex application, it becomes an evolving clinical tool to facilitate new behaviors. Counselors who want to follow theoretical paths and interventions other than family systems theory will use the genogram as a way to gather basic knowledge concerning family members and history.

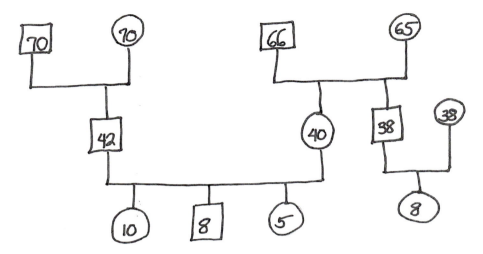

Figure 1.1 Example of genogram with three-generation family

The genogram uses geometric symbols and McGoldrick et al. (2008) have provided a reference that defines universally accepted symbols. Squares usually indicate males and are located on the left; females are on the right represented by circles. Name, birthdate, marriage dates, and death date if applicable are placed near the symbol. Other information such as employment, health history, and cultural factors can be placed near the symbol representing the family member. Lines showing family connections with slashes indicate divorces and other types of connections and separations.

Counselors who use this process with clients will begin to ask questions of the client and begin to map out family relationships such as the one in Figure 1.1 demonstrates by gathering information about marriage dates, births, divorces, and other important family milestones. Counselors who use genograms will apply many types of symbols and lines to indicate relationship disconnects and alliances. Once again, this method of assessing a family can be used in a simple, straightforward manner or in a more complicated therapeutic fashion, all depending on how extensively the counselor wants to use the process.

THE STRATEGIC APPROACH

The Strategic approach to family counseling, founded by Jay Haley and Don Jackson, will take as little information about family history as possible. Instead this approach will want to know more about the specific problem as presented by the family and look at the function of the problem as it relates to the system. Counselors who work from this approach will review the nature of the family concern or problem and ask questions about its impact on individual family members. This type of therapy starts off by gathering information about the family problem, then moves to negotiating a solvable problem, and then works on discovering social situations that make it necessary (Haley, 1987). Strategic therapy requires the therapist to take a directive stance with primary responsibility for understanding the problem and developing an effective intervention. The task for the family therapist is to design interventions that will interrupt current dysfunctional patterns (Haley, 1986) The strategic family counselor will identify a solvable problem, design an intervention, and review the outcomes of the intervention to allow for redesigning the applied plan. Basic techniques in this process involve interviewing, observation, and analysis. Therapists take a proactive direct role in designing strategies that will help families to get out of old patterns and develop new more functional ways of dealing with life.

Sometimes a team approach is used in this therapy, with therapy taking place in a facility that uses a one-way mirror. Teams of therapists will view the live session behind the mirror and offer insight and observation to the counselor in the room (Madanes, 1984). Counselors will use questions in first sessions to ask about what is happening in the family and focus on feedback loops and family patterns that set up the homeostasis, or the status quo, of dysfunctional behaviors. The team of therapists will often make a telephone call in to the counselor in the room and offer directions or suggestions to the counselor or clients.

THE STRUCTURAL APPROACH

The Structural approach, created by Salvador Minuchin, will focus on family patterns and interactions in a similar way as the strategic model by helping to design new ways for the family to interact. Structural family therapy explores family structure, subsystems, and boundaries (Nichols & Davis, 2017). Structural approach to family therapy includes three steps: (1) the therapist joins the family as a leader, (2) discovers family structure, and (3) creates the circumstances that facilitate change in the family structure (Minuchin, 1974, p. 111). One of the ways that structural family therapists would analyze patterns of interaction involved mapping family structure. The therapist would evaluate the family concerning family boundaries. Sometimes families were rated as disengaged or enmeshed (Minuchin, 1974, p. 54). Another way to say it would be that structural therapists identify the family as operating in a function that is too close or too distant for healthy interactions.

Other symbols indicate coalitions among family members, conflict, over involvement, and symbols for enmeshment, to name just a few.

Structural therapy identifies boundary issues as a potential source of family dysfunction. Minuchin (1974) sees that boundaries must be clear to enable family members to carry out family functions. Structural therapy analyzes family structure and function by classifying members into subsystems. These subsystems can be made up of parents and children, or a situation where a mother aligns with a child against her husband. The mother would be classified as having enmeshed or unclear boundaries with the child and disengaged boundaries with her husband symbolized as in Figure 1.3.

Symbols used in structural family mapping:

_____I_ _ _ _ _ _ _ _ _ _ _ _ _I................

disengaged   clear boundaries   enmeshed

Figure 1.2 Example of lines used in Minuchin's family mapping process

Mother............Child

———————————

Father

The dotted line symbolizes enmeshment and the solid line indicates disengaged.

Figure 1.3 Example of family mapping

Mapping family interactions helps the counselor to understand family interactions and encourages the family to view family problems as expanded to the system versus residing in one individual family member. The family map helps the counselor design a plan of action. More recent applications of structural family therapy see assessment as more than just a possibility of gathering information but as a chance for active dynamic opportunities for ongoing examinations of looking at the way the family perceives the problem. In addition, assessment begins challenging the underlying systemic contributions to the problem. Assessment includes a four-step process that (1) broadens family problem to include context, (2) identifies interactions that maintain the problem, (3) structurally focuses on explorations of the past, and (4) develops a shared vision for future change (Nichols & Tafuri, 2013).

THE EXPERIENTIAL MODEL

The Experiential model of family counseling is credited to Virginia Satir and Carl Whitaker. This model of intervention promotes the concepts of self-actualization and self-expression in family therapy. Emotional suppression is seen as the root of family dysfunction (Nichols & Davis, 2017). This model encourages emotional expression and authenticity (Whitaker, 1976). Experiential therapy processes family member's emotional experiences versus a focus on structure of the family and problem-solving. Experiential family interventions focus on getting to know family members, and counselors will ask individuals in the family to describe the family and to express information about experiences in the here and now. Satir, Stachowiak, and Taschman (1976) focused on feelings within families and helped family members to get a sense of what it was like to be a person in the family.

Some experiential family counselors will use expressive techniques such as family sculpture, where family members are arranged in representative positions to portray family experience (Duhl, Kanto, & Duhl, 1973). Other techniques involve the use of conjoint family drawings, where family members are able to draw themselves as they see themselves as a group (Bing, 1970). Utilizing art as a psychotherapeutic technique helps the family to express feelings all at the same time, potentially uncovering unconscious feelings (Kwiatkowska, 1967). Other expressive family art measures include the symbolic drawing of the family life space, a technique that is considered a projective technique (Nichols & Swartz, 1995). In addition to using drawings and family art, expressive tools and techniques include the use of role-playing and family puppets (Nichols & Davis, 2017). Family mapping and graphic techniques are considered tools for family assessment (Thomlison, 2016). Using these expressive tools and interventions can be useful for qualitative family assessment measures (Deacon & Piercy, 2001).

One of the more widely used graphic and visual techniques is the *ecomap* developed by Hartman (1978) as a process to help social workers and other counselors to visually express the relationships between a family and its social environment. The process of the ecomap also uses symbols to represent the individual within the context of the person's family, taking into account social and environmental factors. The ecomap also uses symbols such as circles to indicate the factors relevant to the person's psychosocial situation. At present, many software packages exist to help counselors to diagram the client and the client's social network.

However, the process originally was created as a paper-and-pencil process and was completed often with the interaction of the client. The process design allows counselors to complete the ecomap after interviewing the client or guide the client with information to enable the client to complete the diagram all by themselves. The process of drawing the ecomap involves drawing a center circle and identifying it as the client. Additional circles are drawn around the center circle and can be drawn in sizes relative to the degree of influence that each component asserts on the center circle. After drawing the outside circles the person will symbolically represent connections and relationships to the outside circles by drawing lines that indicate strong connections or tenuous, difficult, or strenuous relationships. Social workers and counselors use the ecomap process as a visual way to understand the individual client situation. The application of the drawing can be used in assessment, getting to know the client, and as a tool to help clients explore systemic relationships. It has also been used as a research tool in discovering social support networks (Ray, 2005). Once again, the depth and use of the tool is left to how the counselor chooses to apply the knowledge gained in completing the process. Hartman (2003, p. 43) reflected on the use of the process as a postmodern tool that helps therapists and clients to be collaborative and client centered.

Despite having wide usage, the ecomap does not have much research related to the process, with the exception of a graduate student study. Calix (2004) developed a project to quantify the ecomap and compare it to other measures of social support. The study was able to show some connections between number of people in the ecomap along with strong or weak connections. These kinds of visual tools present difficulties in developing research studies due to client-specific qualities and lack of numerical components.

PSYCHODYNAMIC FAMILY THERAPY

The psychodynamic model of family therapy was developed by Freudian psychiatrists Nathan Ackerman, Henry Dicks, and Ivan Boszormenyi-Nagy. Psychodynamic therapy utilizes concepts developed by Freud and explores individual drives and developmental tasks. Attention is given to projections and regressions made by the client. Nichols and Davis (2017, p. 160) indicate that psychodynamic family therapists primarily use listening, analytic neutrality, empathy, and interpretations as the basic therapeutic technique. Psychodynamic therapies (Atkeson, 1980) will use assessment in a number of ways that include diagnostic interviews, to review individual issues; family interviews, to focus on possible resistance; family conferences, to provide interpretations; and family group therapy and treatment collaborations, to set up treatment interventions.

Ackerman (1962) shares that psychoanalysis revealed the role of family conflict as a contributor to the development of mental illness. For Ackerman, it was a logical jump to work with families to help alleviate the mental health issues. Ackerman (1962, p. 304) states that a therapeutic approach to emotional disturbances must begin with a psychosocial evaluation of the family as a whole. Other attention has to be concerned with social and educational concerns that might be influencing family disturbances. Psychodynamic models of family assessment ask questions and look for ways to uncover underlying thoughts and

INTRODUCING METHODS OF FAMILY ASSESSMENT | 9

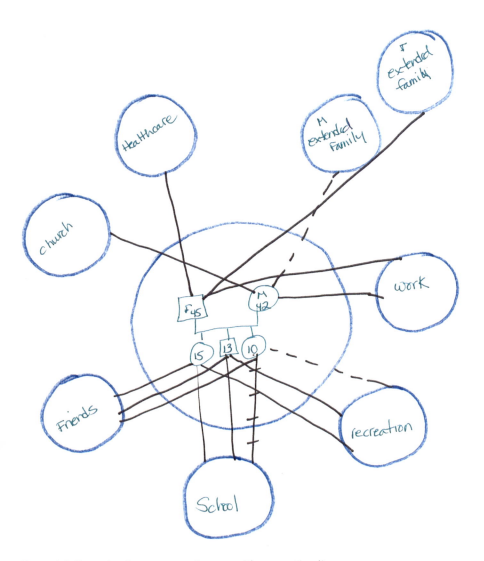

Figure 1.4 Example of an ecomap diagram with connection lines

actions. Ackerman (1962) suggests that psychodynamic family therapy involves focusing on intrapsychic and interpersonal events, unconscious and conscious experiences, unreal and real, transference and reality, past and present, and individual and group. Psychodynamic family therapy will utilize Freudian drive theory, self-psychology, and object relations theory. Nichols and Davis (2017) indicate that object relations theory is the bridge between individual aspects of psychoanalytic focus and recognition that individuals form concepts through connections with significant others. Nichols and Davis (2017, p. 166) reflect that psychodynamic family therapists all agree that the drives within the individual manifest the problem and that symptoms are evidenced and treated in the family context.

Cognitive Behavioral Family Therapy

Cognitive behavioral family therapy orientation to family assessment and treatment is rooted in behavior modification theories and practices (Patterson, 1971). Problematic symptoms are viewed in terms of positive and negative reinforcers (Nichols & Davis, 2017). The social learning approach informs that behaviors can be improved by adding positive outcomes (Stuart, 1980). Behavioral interventions were combined with thought processes to develop interventions that explore behaviors and cognitions. Cognitive behavioral therapy bases interventions on the idea that the best way to change beliefs is through cognitive restructuring, rational analysis, and behavioral enactments (Friedburg, 2006, p. 160).

Assessment seeks to understand how the behavior was initially learned and ingrained. Thoughts and perceptions about the situation are identified and possibly challenged as the therapy proceeds. Dattilio and Freeman (2007) see cognitive behavioral therapy as a circular procession that involves cognitions that evoke emotions and behaviors, which then evoke cognitions. Assessment needs to understand how families develop a sense of self, others, the world, and relationships (Dattilio & Freeman, 2007). These schemas can be drawn out on paper with words and arrows to help families understand and break patterns that do not work for them.

Cognitive behavioral family therapy will often use a structured assessment process that include detailed questionnaires. Sometimes counselors exploring marital relationships will use questionnaires such as the Locke Wallace Marital Adjustment scale (Locke & Wallace, 1959) or scales like the Dyadic Adjustment Scale (Spanier, 1976). Behavioral assessment ratings for children can also be utilized by family counselors along with behavioral checklists to understand family interactions (Nurse & Sperry, 2012). The family counselor will utilize questioning and interviewing to address family belief systems. Nichols and Davis (2017, p. 180) identify steps that a cognitive behavioral assessment will include: (a) identifying family patterns and identifying conflicts inherent in the conflict, (b) tracing origins of the problem, (c) identifying the need for change, (d) enlisting family members in the need for change, (e) assessing ability to make change, (f) implementing new behaviors, and (g) enacting new behaviors along with reinforcing the changes. Cognitive behavioral family assessment identifies the stimulus of the family problem and the reinforcing behaviors that keep it in place, and then begins to challenge current behaviors to create new more functioning behaviors. The final steps involve developing new behaviors and reinforcing supports that will keep the new behavior in operation.

Cognitive behavioral assessment can include observation and surveys. One such measure is the Circumplex Model of Family Assessment. David Olson (2000) developed the Circumplex Model of Marital and Family Systems in an effort to develop a way to systematically classify families and "bridge a gap" between theory and practice and research in treatment. The process ultimately presents a pictorial representation of the family and places the family in terms of functioning on a graph that illustrates family functioning. The model looks at measures related to family cohesion, flexibility, and communication. The model obtains information from self-report surveys, Family Adaptability and Cohesion Evaluation Scale (FACES) and is able to categorize family functioning after obtaining scores from the FACES survey. Olson developed six scales to test relationship cohesion and flexibility (Olson, 2011). The survey has been developed into at least three forms of the measure. Olson reports that families that score at either end of the measure are going to be demonstrating problems. Olson looks for healthy family functioning in scores that are located in the central portion of his scale.

The scale is usually drawn as a circle subdivided into four quadrants. Families who score on the outsides of the quadrants are described as families with problems. The chart describes the categories and indicates that the healthiest families are located in the middle of the chart.

The Olson model collects information from the clients themselves and sometimes has outside observers score the family members. The FACES IV has showed reliability in all scales, and Olson (2011) proposes that the scale be used as a research process.

Solution-Focused Family Therapy

Solution-focused family therapy offers a unique perspective on family intervention by focusing on desired outcomes and goals. Often family therapy focuses on problems versus desired outcomes. This method of treatment asks the clients in the assessment process to define how the family will be different after successful completion of the intervention. This therapy starts by asking clients how the result is supposed to look (Nichols & Davis, 2017). In other words, the beginning starts with defining the positive outcome. Assessment includes defining the problem versus a review of family dynamics or investigations of family constellations. Family history is not as important. The only people that need to be in session are family members who want to do something about the concern that brought people to therapy. Usually this type of therapy needs very little intake information. The early phases of treatment involve exploring possibilities and client's visions for desired results. After utilizing many questions, therapists work to empower clients as the masters of coping with their issues and creators of therapeutic goals. Solution-focused therapy recognizes that there are always exceptions to problem situations and that clients have the solutions to their situations (Visser, 2013).

Solution-focused therapy will collaboratively set up goals and assess progress toward achieving goals by sometimes using number scales that range from 1, a problem at its worst, to 10, where the problem has been eliminated.

The identification of solutions and scales that measure progress toward therapeutic outcome operate along behavioral modification techniques (Nichols & Davis, 2017, pp. 223–224).

The founders of this type of therapy worked with other modes of family therapy and developed their methods as a way of expanding desired outcomes for clients. Steve de Shazer and Insoo Kim Berg are credited with originating this model of intervention. Others that focus on client outcomes and research toward effective solution-oriented treatment include therapists such as Scott Miller and Michelle Weiner-Davis (Visser, 2013).

(worst)1----------------------------------10 (goal achieved)

Figure 1.5 Solution-focused therapy progress scale

Narrative Family Therapy

The final model of family therapy for this introductory review is narrative family therapy. Narrative family therapy focuses on social constructionist and constructionist approaches to social change and takes into account how language sets up and maintains the problem (Etchison & Kleist, 2000). This model of family therapy takes family experience as constructed and given specific meaning by the people involved in the family. Narrative therapy maintains that therapists cannot just observe the family to understand what is going on, and that intervention requires interacting with family members to understand their own experiences and interpretations. Narrative therapy would find it very important to know more about the client's understanding and the story that the client has of themselves. These messages involve cultural and societal narratives. Narrative therapists focus on internal messages versus looking to solve problems. Interventions often externalize the message of cultural and societal assumptions to allow clients to free themselves from these old tapes and stories. A key intervention involves externalizing the problem by asking questions that deconstruct the problems to facilitate mastery over it.

Narrative family therapy likes to obtain information about how the family perceives their story and their experience with the problem. Nichols & Davis (2017) identifies the narrative therapist as both an anthropologist and a hypnotist. Questions are utilized that both empower clients to identify and see problems in a new way. White (1995) encourages therapists who work with him on a reflecting team to let go of theorizing about the truth of problems that clients bring. Therapists are encouraged to be attentive to the current discussions and avoid the stance of other family therapies that might focus on preparing interventions or problem-solving or offering advice.

Family assessment involves the use of mapping the influence of the problem on the family along with recognizing the influence of the family on the problem. Questions might involve

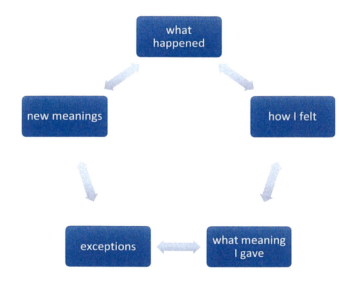

Figure 1.6 Example of narrative problem mapping process

identifying what happened to create the presenting concern. Follow-up questions ask the client about how they felt in that situation and what meaning they applied to the issue. Important follow-up questions tap into the client's own resources and ask about times when the client behaved differently. Counselors then pursue ideas on how new meanings can be applied to the situation. The mapping process involves seeing the problem but also recognizing exceptions to the problem and how the family has demonstrated strength in managing the problem. White (2007) uses maps to help clients find new ways to perceive themselves and their circumstances.

Common Components of Family Assessment

Reviewing the various models of family therapy, it is easy to see that the type of model the therapist operates from will have a lot to do with the way that the family will be assessed. Despite the various orientations to family therapy, most therapists have developed an integrative and eclectic approach to providing family services (Nichols & Swartz, 2008). Therapists will develop and learn a basic model and expand their understanding of family structure and ways to intervene with clients. Agencies and state regulations often call for collection of information that does not necessarily fit some of the treatment orientations. An example would be if a therapist or counselor wanted to follow a narrative approach and would not want to obtain a lot of history that an agency might require in an intake process.

Some models such as Bowen's will want to focus on the whole family, while other models focus on individual experience. Models such as structural therapy will look for behaviors and sequences of behaviors that create or maintain symptoms (Nichols & Tafuri, 2013). Postmodern models do not focus on family dynamics or history but look for ideas and concepts that facilitate symptom relief and solutions. Cognitive behavioral approaches will develop scales or client self-report measures that add in tracking progress.

Sperry (2012) reports that family assessment involves different categories of measuring the client situation that include qualitative, standardized, observational, ongoing assessment, and self-report measures. Qualitative measures include unstructured interviewing, role-playing, and graphic methods like the genogram. Use of interviewing seems to be the most commonly used method of assessment in most treatment models. Standardized assessments include surveys and scales that have been tested for validity and reliability. Observational measures record and systematically chart behaviors and observations. Ongoing assessment such as outcome rating scales (ORS) can provide information on outcomes and can offer a structured process that is referenced often or weekly in the counseling process (Duncan, 2010). Self-report measures are often used in client assessment to report on a client's felt sense of experience. These measures are quick and help the client and counselor know how the therapy is being experienced in the here and now. Most models of family therapy use one or more of these types of assessment categories.

Counselors have the opportunity to use many processes for family assessment. The various models and therapy orientations provide direction on how to utilize the various tools available toward effective family assessment. Thomlison (2016) indicates that the various tools for assessment include interviewing techniques, mapping and graphic techniques, time lines, family scales, and observational techniques. As previously noted, interviewing and questioning is a key component of family assessment and is commonly used in all orientations. Therapists may or may not follow specific guidelines as to the questions asked of family members. The interview can be part of information gathering or it can be applied to the interventions utilized in family sessions. Mapping and graphic devices provide visual tools for family members to understand family structure and patterns. The genogram and ecomap both provide visuals of family history and involvement with social structures in the outside world. Time lines are also visual opportunities to trace family events. Family scales make use of the standardized surveys that provide information about individual and family functioning. Observational techniques have the evaluator watching families as they work on a joint project or enact a family situation. All of these tools can be taken at face value, or information gathered can be utilized to implement interventions. Many of the tools can be used in an integrated practice of family treatment.

Purpose and Value of Family Assessment

Despite the various theoretical approaches to treating families, some common rationales appear as contributing to the desirability of the assessment process. According to Ghanbaripanah and Mustaffa (2012), family assessment can provide information related to: family process, family affect, family organization, experience and history of the problem, and family strengths. Williams, Edwards, Patterson, and Chamow (2011, pp. 34–43) add that family assessment can provide information concerning client goals, expectations for therapy, and insight into client motivation and past attempted solutions. Regardless of the therapeutic model or theoretical orientation, family assessment helps provide the therapist with some direction and orientation toward the next steps in therapy. Most agencies and organizations require some attention to identify client information and create checklists for identifying clients and treatment paths.

Families can be assessed by reviewing factors related to a holistic review of the family situation (Patterson, Williams, Edwards, Chamow, & Grauf-Grounds, 2009, p. 67). This holistic review includes the biological situation, psychological factors, family systems, psychosocial information, ethnic and cultural concerns, social issues, and spiritual considerations. Effective family assessment will take into account all the factors affecting the family. While exploring basic information about members of the family, the counselor also needs to be aware of risk factors affecting family members. Risk factors include issues related to basic needs along with concerns of substance abuse and domestic violence. Special recognition needs to be in place that all family members are functioning in a multilayered system and having individual as well as collective experiences. Assessment is not always an easy process, and assessment tools need to be mindful of the complicated issues facing family groups.

Family assessment provides not only an opportunity for specifying identifying information about the family, but it can be a therapeutic tool as well. Assessment establishes a baseline for treatment that tracks progress and helps families to expand current insight into their situation as treatment evolves (Deacon & Piercy, 2001). Evaluating the family allows therapist and client alike to have a sense of direction and ideas as to what everyone is looking for in terms of a successful outcome. Most family therapy interventions seem to operate around some common principles for change and can include a planned systematic approach, involvement of the whole family, recognition of family members' expertise about themselves, and therapist attention to evidence-based practices (Thomlison, 2016). Family assessment is an opportunity to know the client, understand family dynamics, and figure out where to go, and to discover if the treatment process actually provided a valuable experience along the way.

CRUCIAL QUALITIES OF EFFECTIVE ASSESSMENT

No matter the model or orientation approach to working with families, a key necessary concept emerges as a crucial factor in effective treatment. Therapists need to form a connection with the clients they serve. Patterson et al. (2009) and Williams et al. (2011) underscore the need for joining clients in the early stages of treatment. Clients want to know that the counselor cares about them and knows the issues that affect them. Most clients like to share their story and concerns when seeking consultations with mental health providers. Thomlison (2016) identifies the process of developing an alliance as one of the common factors in successful family outcomes. Developing an alliance with each member of the family will be a key factor in the future outcome of treatment. Most treatment models identify developing an alliance as the skill that set the stage for successful therapy (Nichols & Davis, 2017).

Therapists and counselors who are able to engage and explore family issues with clients will have the opportunity to work more effectively with clients. Wampold (2015) shares that the common factors that have positive impact on effective psychotherapy outcome are developing an alliance, a sense of empathy, a sense of expectations, cultural adaptations of evidence-based treatments, and therapist effect. Wampold (2015) notes that clients often make very rapid decisions about their willingness to engage in the therapeutic relationship and that first sessions are very important, as clients often will not continue counseling after one session. Sundet (2011) indicates that clients considered the relationship helpful and collaborative when they were listened to, taken seriously, and allowed to follow their own goals and ideas.

Elements of effective joining and developing good alliances with clients in initial sessions include asking questions, listening with curiosity, showing understanding, and offering nonjudgmental reflections. The skills that facilitate joining can be developed, but it has to be noted that developing an effective counseling relationship is not something that can be formulated by using a technique (Patterson et al., 2009). Therapist factors such as personality, style and their own reactivity to certain situations affect the joining process.

Initial family assessments are designed to help the client and therapist to find some way to organize and understand the process of treatment. Most family therapy assessment concerns some way of defining the problem, setting goals and expectations for therapy, and understanding client motivation and attempted past solutions (Thomlison, 2016). Assessments involve understanding strengths and resources as well as understanding factors involving personal reactions of the therapist. Therapists have a wide array of tools and techniques to utilize in understanding family dynamics and focus of treatment. Effective family therapy will be aware of engaging clients on their own terms and of creating an atmosphere of mutual respect. Therapists need to be able to connect with clients as they engage in the initial treatment process.

THE FAMILY LIFE SPACE DRAWING

Flash back to our family in the counseling waiting room, who meets with a counselor and shares their first session and counseling assessment through the Family Life Space Drawing (FLSD). The FLSD is a graphic assessment process that includes all members of the family system in representing visually the current family dynamics. It is an opportunity to include all family members in the assessment process at the same time. The FLSD provides information about family members and describes intergenerational issues in the same way as the genogram but with a hands-on, client-originated process. Additional information about family relationships and connection comes from the process of placing the symbols in the content of the family drawing. The FLSD provides information about the environmental stressors related to all of the family members – much in the way that the ecomap process describes, but in a common space. The value of the FLSD over the ecomap is that the clients are able to potentially provide unconscious information related to spatial and size placement of the symbols. The clients place symbols themselves at their own direction versus following a structured placement process controlled by the counselor or therapist. The FLSD does not provide a categorization of families in the manner of a survey or observational process such as the Circumplex Model of Family Assessment. However, the FLSD has the potential to allow clients and counselor to have a process whereby each gets to know the other and form a process for developing goals for treatment.

The family will have an opportunity to share information in an interactive, physically expressive manner as they symbolically share information about each family member's backgrounds. In addition, each family member receives individual attention and time to express their perspectives and environmental factors. Any family member who is not comfortable with verbal disclosure has the opportunity to share symbolically and nonverbally.

The FLSD model has the potential for obtaining information that other assessment models provide and so much more. The time that it takes to conduct the FLSD can be completed in one session. Many clients report that the process of completing the FLSD conveyed more information in a shorter time than they had ever expressed in previous counseling sessions. The process of conducting the session and gathering information is easy and can quickly help counselors and clients to see and assess treatment and counseling needs.

The FLSD can be taken at face value as a way to get acquainted with clients and to systematically develop a joining tool of interacting with clients, conveying a sense of interest and respect. In addition to using the process on that simple level, counselors can potentially explore other levels of information that the FLSD provides. Placement of the symbols creates opportunities for curiosity and questions that help facilitate the relationship between clients and counselors or therapists. The FLSD assessment measure helps counselors who desire to use a process that informs systemically on the family and, at the same time, it helps to create a therapeutic alliance and develop treatment goals and desired treatment outcomes.

The family life space drawing process is a way to accomplish the traditionally desired goals of family assessment that include knowing family organization, structure, and family strengths. The process provides individual reflections of the problem, strengths, a need for resources, and spiritual influences past and present. Co-creating the FLSD process provides information about family functioning, communication patterns, and current stresses affecting each member. Perhaps the most valuable aspect of conducting the family life space drawing process is the opportunity to develop an effective alliance with individual family members. Conducting the process of the FLSD allows the therapist to listen with interest, genuine humanity, and empathy. Interviewing and listening skills are combined through the vehicle of the visual graphic experience to give family members a sense that the therapist counselor knows them through the completion of the process. The process is a collaborative event and can be applied to any model of intervention. As Wampold (2015) notes, the model of intervention is not as important as the client-therapist relationship. Completing the interactive process allows for the first step of client therapist engagement that can follow any applied therapeutic path.

Families who complete the FLSD process will have an opportunity to complete a qualitative, graphic measure with the counselor or therapist. Therapists will use interviewing and questioning skills as the process ensues. The process will be client centered and obtain information about family components, structures, and background information. Clients are able to identify stressors, risk factors, and biopsychosocial elements affecting their family. Most importantly, the process facilitates the client and therapist relationship as they develop treatment goals and future plans for the therapeutic process. The family leaves the session with a sense of relief, knowing that the counselor connects to who they are and what they are facing. They have all had personalized attention and opportunity to express their individual perspectives and provide insight on analyzing the drawing for what it might report. All of the family members have had an opportunity to reflect on treatment needs and goals. Clients experience the session with a sense of being heard and respected with confidence that the therapist will work with them toward common goals. In short, the family leaves with less anxiety and a concrete sense that the counseling sessions will provide value to the family.

Summary

There are many theories and orientations to provide interventions with families. Some interventions are interested in family history, while other interventions like to focus on the here and now of the presenting situation. All the orientations require some sense of assessment or engagement with the family. Assessment has some common features, such as taking time to join the family to develop some rapport or trust, even if the theory does not require an interest in obtaining family history. Developing an alliance or connection to the family is a crucial component of the family therapy process, no matter the orientation or theoretical approach to assisting the family. The FLSD is an effective tool for developing the connection process with the client and developing an effective alliance, whatever the theoretical approach might be in working with the family. The FLSD can obtain history if that is a desired goal, but it does not have to focus on that issue. The greatest value of the FLSD is in addressing the concerns and thoughts of all family members in one space and in one assessment session. It is a useful tool for all theoretical orientations that work with families.

References

Ackerman, N. (1962). Family psychotherapy and psychoanalysis: The implications of difference Family Process, 1, 30–43.
Atkeson, P. (1980). The psychodynamic approach to family therapy. In S. Priester & D. Sollee (Eds.), *Family change theory: Family therapy*. Volume II of Resources in Family Studies. Washington, DC: The Catholic University of America.
Bing, E. (1970). The conjoint family drawing. *Family Process*, 9, 173–194.
Bowen, M. (1978). *Family therapy in clinical practice*. New York, NY: Jason Aronson.
Calix, A. R. (2004). *Is the ecomap a valid and reliable social work tool to measure social support?* Master thesis. Baton Rouge, LA: Louisiana State University.
Dattilio, F. M. & Freeman, A. (2007). Introduction. In F. M. Dattilio & A. Freeman (Eds.), *Cognitive-behavioral strategies in crisis intervention*. New York, NY: Guildford Press.
Deacon, S. A., & Piercy, F. P. (2001). Qualitative methods in family evaluation: Creative assessment techniques. *American Journal of Family Therapy*, 29(5), 355–373.

Duhl, F. J., Kanto, D., & Duhl, B. S. (1973). Learning space and action in family therapy: A Primer of sculpture. In D. A. Bloch (Ed.), *Techniques of family therapy*. New York, NY: Grune & Stratton.

Duncan, B. L. (2010). *On becoming a better therapist*. Washington, DC: American Psychological Association.

Etchison, M., & Kleist, D. M. (2000). Review of narrative therapy: Research and utility. *The Family Journal: Counseling and Therapy for Couples and Families*, 8(1), 61–66.

Fogarty, T. F. (1976). Systems concepts and the dimensions of self. In P. Guerin (Ed.), *Family Therapy: Theory and practice*. New York, NY: Gardner Press.

Friedburg, R. D. (2006). A cognitive-behavioral approach to family therapy. *Journal of Contemporary Psychotherapy*, 36, 159–165. https://doi.org/10.1007/s10879-006-9020-2

Ghanbaripanah, A., & Mustaffa, M. S. (2012). The review of family assessment in counseling. *International Journal of Fundamental Psychology & Social Sciences*, 2(2), 32–35.

Haley, J. (1986). *Uncommon therapy*. New York, NY: W. W. Norton & Company.

Haley, J. (1987). *Problem solving therapy* (2nd ed.). San Francisco, CA: Jossey-Bass.

Hartman, A. (1978). Diagrammatic assessment of family relationships. *Social Casework*, 59, 465–476.

Hartman, A. (2003). Comments on diagrammatic assessment of family relations. *Reflections*, summer, 41–44.

Kerr, M., & Bowen, M. (1988). *Family evaluation*. New York, NY: W. W. Norton & Co.

Locke, H. J., & Wallace, K. M. (1959). Short term marital adjustment and prediction tests: Their reliability and validity. *Marriage and Family Living*, 21, 251–255.

Madanes, C. (1984). *Behind the one way mirror: Advances in the practice of strategic therapy*. San Francisco, CA: Jossey-Bass.

McGoldrick, M., Gerson, R., & Petry, S. (2008). *Genograms: Assessment and interventions* (3rd ed.). New York, NY: W. W. Norton & Company.

Minuchin, S. (1974). *Families and family therapy*. Cambridge, MA: Harvard University Press.

Nichols, M. P., & Davis, S. D. (2017). *Family therapy: Concepts and methods* (11th ed.). Boston, MA: Pearson.

Nichols, M. P., & Swartz, R. C. (1995). *Family therapy: Concepts and methods* (3rd ed.). Boston, MA: Pearson.

Nichols, M. P., & Swartz, R. C. (2008). *Family therapy: Concepts and methods* (8th ed.). Boston, MA: Pearson.

Nichols, M. P., & Tafuri, S. (2013). Techniques of structural family assessment: A qualitative Analysis of how experts promote a systemic perspective. *Family Process*, 52(2), 207–215. https://doi.org/10.1111/famp.12025

Nurse, A. R., & Sperry, L. (2012). Standardized assessment. In L. Sperry (Ed.), *Family assessment: Contemporary and cutting edge strategies* (2nd ed.). New York, NY: Taylor & Francis Group.

Olson, D. H. (2000). Circumplex model of family systems. *Journal of Family Therapy*, 22(2), 144–167.

Olson, D. H. (2011). FACES IV and the circumplex model: Validation study. *Journal of Marital and Family Therapy*, 37(1), 64–80 https://doi.org/10.1111/j.1752-0606.2009.00175x

Patterson, G. R. (1971). *Families: Applications of social learning to family life*. Champaign, IL: Research Press.

Patterson, J., Williams, L., Edwards, T., Chamow, L., & Grauf-Grounds, C. (2009). *Essential skills in family therapy: From first interview to termination*. New York, NY: Guildford Press.

Ray, R. A. (2005). Ecomapping: An innovative research tool for nurses. *Journal of Advanced Nursing*, 50(5), 545–552. https://doi.org/10.11vj1365.2005.03431

Satir, V., Stachowiak, J., & Taschman, A. (1976). *Helping families to change*. New York, NY: Jason Aronson Inc.

Spanier, G. B. (1976). Measuring dyadic adjustment: New scales for assessing the quality of marriage and similar dyads. *Journal of Marriage and the Family*, 38, 15–28.

Sperry, L. (2012). Family assessment an overview. In L. Sperry (Ed.), *Family assessment: Contemporary and cutting edge strategies* (2nd ed.). New York, NY: Taylor Francis Group.

Stuart, R. B. (1980). *Helping couples change*. New York, NY: Guilford Press.

Sundet, R. (2011). Collaboration: Family and therapist perspectives of helpful therapy. *Journal of Marital & Family Therapy, 37*(2), 236–249. https://doi.org/10.1111/j.1752-0606.2009.00157.x

Thomlison, B. (2016). *Family assessment handbook: An introduction to family assessment* (4th ed.). Boston, MA: Cengage Learning.

Visser, C. F. (2013). The origin of solution-focused approach. *International Journal of Solution-Focused Practice, 1*, 1. https://doi.org/10.14335/ijsfp.vlil.10

Wampold, B. (2015). How important are the common factors in psychotherapy? An update. *World Psychiatry, 5*(14), 270–277.

Whitaker, C. (1976). The hindrance of theory in clinical work. In P. J. Guerin (Ed.), *Family therapy: Theory and practice* (pp. 154–164). New York, NY: Gardner Press.

White, M. (1995). *Re-authoring lives: Interviews and essays*. Adelaide: Dulwich Centre Publications. Retrieved from www.dulwichcentre.com.au/reflecting-teamwork-as-definitional-ceremony-michael-white.pdf

White, M. (2007). *Maps of narrative practice*. New York, NY: W. W. Norton & Co.

Williams, L., Edwards, T. M., Patterson, J., & Chamow, L. (2011). *Essential skills for couple and family therapists*. New York, NY: Guilford Press.

CHAPTER TWO
The Family Life Space Drawing: History and Development of the Process

Danuta Mostwin

Changing societal dynamics affecting the post-WWII American family created the foundation for Danuta Mostwin, DSW (1921–2010) to develop a systemic family intervention process to support families of troubled and predelinquent youth. Dr. Mostwin recognized the family as a valuable part of human ecology as important as "air and water" and wanted to develop interventions to help families accomplish the primary task of raising healthy children (Mostwin, 1980b, p. 23). In Mostwin's view, families were having difficulties with navigating family structure and the roles of parenting. Her concerns for the future families made her a passionate and strong advocate for helping families navigate the difficulties of societal changes.

One of the components of her family therapy interventions was the creation of the FLSD as a way to assess and engage the families. The FLSD was developed through the influences of Dr. Mostwin's rich life experiences and education. Dr. Mostwin was born in Poland and originally desired to pursue a life career as a physician. Her educational experiences and life expectations changed dramatically with the invasion of the Nazis into her homeland. While living in Poland, she was involved in the underground resistance and spent many years working with groups to rescue Jews and others away from the Nazis in power at the time. At that point her life would take on the attributes of an action-adventure movie and involved being exposed to troubling and violent situations. After the war ended, she was placed in a difficult position by the occupation of the Soviet Union and was forced both to deny her claim to her educational degree and to leave her homeland to find a new life, which she eventually found in the United States.

In the United States, Mostwin studied social work, eventually obtaining a Master's degree in Social Work from the Catholic University of America and a Doctoral degree in Social Work from Columbia in 1971. Mostwin's early research focused on the impact of ethnicity on the American population and the adjustments of immigrant groups within the United States (Mostwin, 1972). Her work was concerned with cultural and ethnic influences on immigration, and Margaret Mead was her dissertation chair toward that endeavor. The focus of ethnic identity was explored in her research by examining Polish post-WWII immigrants and categorizing their adjustments as they integrated attachments to their homeland and their new country in the United States. Mostwin carried her passion for understanding ethnic influences throughout her career as a professor and encouraged her graduate social work students to explore the roots of their own ethnic identities (Mostwin, 1977a).

While at Columbia, Mostwin was influenced by the rising focus of systems theory and its application to social work practice. The concept of ecological social work practice and awareness of environmental factors versus a singular focus on intrapsychic forces was a predominant concept in the educational experiences of students in the social work program at the time (Germain, 1973). Joining Dr. Mostwin at Columbia as a student was Ann Hartman, the creator of the ecomap, a similar process to the FLSD. Hartman observes that the ecological systems concept was advancing in the academic environment of Columbia during the 1970s. (2003).

Working with a family-centered approach versus an individual focus was an emerging concept at the time of her graduation, and Dr. Mostwin continued her work with a family intervention orientation. Her early social work career included working with the Maryland Children's Aid Society, helping with adoption. Mostwin continued the focus on the impact of ethnicity by continuing to work with immigrant families in the Baltimore region, especially those of Polish, Estonian, Ukrainian, Hungarian, Czechoslovakian, and Lithuanian origins. Her concern for ethnic influences was not only for recent immigrants but also for families who arrived in the United States over a hundred years ago and now called themselves Americans. Mostwin recognized that ethnicity played an important role in family culture even when the family members did not have a conscious connection to their original home place origins. Helping clients and family groups to understand the role that ethnicity played in possible family stress and adjustments became a strong focus of her life's work.

After many years in academia, Mostwin spent the final years of her life focusing on her literary efforts related to novels and historical sagas. Her writings drew critical acclaim for her powerful stories about Polish families and post-WWII adjustments. Her books are still available in several languages, although she wrote primarily in her native Polish. Some of her books were nominated for the Nobel Prize in Literature in 2000 and 2006.

As part of Mostwin's work as a professor at the Catholic University of America, National Catholic School of Social Service (NCSSS) in Washington, DC, she was a faculty coordinator for the Family Studies Center, guiding graduate students. The training involved working with families as a part of clinical practice. Mostwin began to have several students work with one family at a time and observed that having several therapists working with a family became powerfully effective. Mostwin shared her insights of working with multiple therapists in short-term therapy at the annual conference of the Child Welfare League in 1972 and published articles on working with families through a team of therapists for one family (Mostwin, 1974a, 1976a).

The Family Studies Center moved to several locations, but the predominate focus of the center was to train social work students as family therapists. The Family Studies Center also welcomed professionals from other disciplines who were interested in learning more about the practice of family therapy interventions and working with a team approach. Family therapy interventions were a new treatment modality at that time, and many people were interested in learning how to work with families. Mostwin coordinated work with students at the Family Studies Center until 1977 before passing directorship of the program over to Ron Clark, one of her previous students. Dr. Mostwin worked at the Catholic University of America from 1969 to 1980, and then she worked at Loyola College in Baltimore from 1980 to 1987. At both facilities, Dr. Mostwin taught students of social work and mental health in the concepts of family therapy as a treatment intervention.

At both institutions, Dr. Mostwin developed internship programs where students could be trained in hands-on applications of family therapy. She was a strong proponent of using systems theory concepts and trained many students toward the application of using family therapy – then a new and emerging treatment model. Mostwin selected a team of graduate students who wanted to focus on family mental health to work on the family intervention team as early as 1969 (Mostwin, 1977a, p. 51). Her early work in these teaching clinics involved families from lower-middle-class economic levels and various ethnic backgrounds and races. The predominant presenting problem was related to an adolescent family member.

While Mostwin was working with interns and encouraging them to work with clients and their families, she developed the team approach to family intervention. The original experiment in the team approach to family therapy started at Johns Hopkins Hospital, with three social work interns and a psychiatrist along with Dr. Mostwin treating a family, where each family member could have an individual therapist and a combined family treatment experience. The team approach continued to evolve, as the Family Studies Center would select students to join this treatment team, providing individual and a group family therapy experience.

Mostwin organized student and faculty seminars from 1974 to 1982 to provide information on the concepts of family treatment and to advance the multidimensional model of working with families. The treatment focused mostly on delinquent and predelinquent teens. All of these seminars promoted the use of her short-term model of intervention and the use of the FLSD as a way to first meet and understand the families in treatment. In addition to the theoretical influences previously mentioned, Dr. Mostwin included Lewin's field theory, and the work of relational systems thinkers such as Boszormenyi-Nagy and Herbert Mead's symbolic interaction theories, as inspiration for her team approach to family interventions (Mostwin, 1980a). These theoretical influences that form the theoretical foundation of the FLSD will be discussed in later chapters.

Short-Term Multidimensional Family Intervention

Mostwin developed a group approach to working with families that is time limited and oriented to working with a family in crisis. The intervention process was originally called Short-Term Multidimensional Family Intervention (STMFI) (Mostwin, 1980a). Preister (1974, p. 42) informs that the concept of "multidimensional" comes from involving the family in "different modes" of treatment that include group, joint, and individual contacts. He expands the multidimensional concept by recognizing that the therapy focuses on community systems that are important to family success, such as schools, church, employment, and other organizations interacting with the family.

The STMFI process provided a model for working with families in crisis situations where the potential for systems change may be the greatest (Mostwin, 1976b). The intervention worked to address family issues in a quick, task-oriented fashion. The dynamic interfacing action of individual and group therapies were employed as vehicles to address this change. The goals of therapy hoped to invoke the emergent properties of the system, eventually evolving to create the desired outcome of family restructuring that facilitates effective family function.

The STMFI model addressed six dimensions of treatment concerns: spatial dimension, holistic dimension, symbolic interaction, social dimension, cultural dimension, and intrapersonal dimension (Mostwin, 1980a).

Spatial dimension identifies and recognizes the family members and their positions in relation to one another. The spatial dimension also notices family boundaries as being either strong or weak. Environmental factors are identified, such as institutions and community groups and psychological or stress factors, that could be affecting the family or specific individuals within the life space.

Holistic dimension attention views the situation as a whole versus narrowing down the family to its component parts. Mostwin (1980a, p. 11) addresses this concept as taking a bird's-eye view of the family. This view sees the whole of family functioning. Mostwin (1980a) sees the FLSD as a facilitator of viewing the family as a whole.

Symbolic interaction dimension explores the meaning that interactions between family members apply to each other. The process of the FLSD that includes communication lines helps to inform on the experience that family interactions have on specific members of the family. The communication lines help by reinforcing or challenging the therapist's perceptions of family interactions.

Social dimension concerns the interaction of family members with each other and their environmental or institutional components. The social dimension recognizes that the various environmental factors from each person in the family have an impact on the whole of family functions. Focusing on the environmental dynamics as a strength or developing need helps to direct treatment interventions.

Cultural dimensions address the impact of cultural heritage on family functioning. Mostwin expands her interest in culture and ethnicity by exploring a family's cultural background with her family interventions. Families can then develop change processes that support or challenge cultural influence as a way to enhance family function.

The final dimension or focus of treatment involves the recognition that the *intrapersonal dimension* of the individual family members plays an important part in family functioning. While the main focus of Mostwin's multidimensional therapy intervention is the macro system of the family, she recognizes that individual functioning has an impact on the types of situations families may face and interventions that may be applied to helping the family through a crisis-oriented intervention. Individual attention is not the main focus of the multidimensional intervention, but sometimes certain individual developmental areas have to receive attention to improve family functioning.

Mostwin (1976b, p. 83) saw the STMFI model as a time-limited, crisis-oriented team approach that could treat various problem situations facing troubled youth. Mostwin combined the individual approach to therapy – more common at that time period – with the group approach of family treatment. Combining the two orientations and serving as a team member made it easier for individually oriented therapists who joined the teams to experience the process of family work. The family therapy team played an important role in facilitating Mostwin's goal of helping families improve not only interfamilial communication channels but also acting as a bridge that would help the family toward improved communications and connections with community organizations.

Mostwin organized treatment teams to work with families and the teams were intended to cope with the family crisis. The treatment teams usually included graduate students in social work, but as previously noted, the teams also included professionals from the community who might be working with the family in another capacity. Clients were referred by hospitals, social service agencies, and other community organizations. Mostwin attempted to match family members with a therapist who might be similar to them. The oldest member of the family was usually partnered with the oldest member of the family therapy team, matching gender if possible.

The focus of the intervention team was not always the traditional goals of psychotherapy of the time, which often set a goal of intrapsychic change within the individual.

Goals of this treatment process were defined by Mostwin (1976a, p. 8) as:

1. Redefinition of the problem
2. Introducing or correcting family roles
3. Improving or opening family's interaction with community organizations
4. Reestablishing family's sense of autonomy.

The STMFI model usually consists of six sessions of intensive work with the family intervening as a team with the clients in individual and dyadic sessions (Clark, 1980). Mostwin (1980a, p. 54) defines the STMFI model as having treatment procedures that include:

1. Multilevel interventions
2. Time-limited crisis therapy
3. A team of therapists.

Preister (1974, p. 41) informs that the goal of the STMFI model is not intended to resolve underlying problems as defined by traditional therapy interventions, but it is intended to "unlock" the family system in order to develop new forms of communication.

The first family session, which often takes about two hours, is structured or identified in four phases which include:

1. Completion of the symbolic drawing of the family life space;
2. Meeting with family members to individually assign a therapist to a family member;
3. Meeting with family to begin identifying the problem; sometimes the therapist will engage in the alter-ego technique at this time;
4. Negotiating a contract with the family.

The initial session of the STMFI model included the use of the diagnostic process, completing a pictorial image of the family using the FLSD as a symbolic representation of the family. Family members work together under the guidance and direction of the therapists to produce a diagram or picture of the family (Clark, 1980, p. 31). The family life space drawing allows for family members to individually identify their sense of the problem or crisis facing the family. Therapist team members meet and reflect on observations as to what the drawing might mean to individuals within the family and the system as a whole. These observations are shared with the whole family.

The remaining sessions of weeks two through five follow similar formats of meeting as a family therapist group with individual sessions followed by family sessions. Session two clarifies and clearly defines family goals developed by team and family members. Each week, the time-limited nature of the treatment is emphasized, with the therapist team leader often reminding everyone of the sessions completed and how many sessions might be left in the treatment contract. The therapist may say something like: "This is week two; we have four sessions left." The team acts in a directive dynamic way, often assigning specific tasks for family members to complete between sessions.

The final session of the STMFI model also includes completing the family life space drawing. The week one drawing and the week six drawings are reviewed and shared with the family as a way to note changes that might have occurred in the process of treatment. After completing 6 weeks of working with the family, the therapists write letters to the whole family and to specific members of the family. Each member receives their own copy. The team makes suggestions and recommendations in the letter and sets up an appointment with the family to meet them in their home after another six-week interval. The last meeting with the team and family takes place after a six-week break, during which there are no meetings and no contact with the therapist team. The home visit is designed to celebrate family progress and to recognize their mastery of the family problem (Clark, 1980, p. 42). Therapists are encouraged to allow the family space to regroup and develop their own coping and management skills without therapist intervention during the six-week break.

Sometimes family members continue counseling treatment with other professionals after the team treatment has completed, but the goal of therapy is to set emergent parts of the system to operate in a new way. The STMFI process is intended to stabilize a family crisis and set up new ways of family functioning that mobilize their own resources and strengths (Mostwin, 1980a, p. 212). The time-limited nature of the intervention was intended to place pressure on the family to reorganize in the fastest way possible.

The STMFI model involves many methods of intervening with families and can include various processes and techniques. Mostwin (1980a, pp. 54–55) also informs that the techniques of treatment involve:

1. Symbolic drawing of the family
2. Setting goals
3. Assigning tasks
4. Therapists acting as alter egos
5. Engaging in play therapy
6. Restructuring the family system
7. Reaching across family boundaries
8. Having a multigenerational perspective
9. Writing letters to the family
10. Following up with a home visit.

The team of therapists often used the technique of acting as an alter-ego partner for the individual family members. The technique of the alter ego as practiced in STMFI has a similarity to the auxiliary ego from psychodrama but differs in that the STMFI alter ego is sympathetic and identifies with the client and models appropriate interactions (Medway & Geddes, 1976). When STMFI team members work together as alter egos, they can interact with each other, demonstrating to each counterpart ways to make communication work more effectively. The team therapist, with permission from the client, assumes the role of the client when they seem stuck, afraid or unable to speak for themselves. When representing the client, the therapist speaks on their behalf, expressing perceived thoughts, opinions, feeling, desires, longings, and other expressions unspoken from the client. The therapist will then check back with the client to question as to how faithfully they represented the client's unspoken experience (Banning & Zinni, 1980) inform that the process of using the alter ego by therapists has the following steps:

1. Focusing on the client's inner thoughts and feelings
2. Rephrasing something the client has said
3. Voicing the words of the client
4. Offering support and encouragement
5. Acknowledging a client's verbal or nonverbal response
6. Representing, or taking the place of an absent family member in session.

The STMFI model was designed to provide a conceptual model for viewing the family as a social system bound by ties of symbolic interaction. It was also designed to provide training to students of family mental health. Last but by no means least, the model was intended to treat families especially those families in crisis (Mostwin, Clark, Depenbrock, McKee, & Picado, 1977). Students of Mostwin and Clark have used this model in organizations and agencies all over the world. Acting as Mostwin's representative, Clark took this model to Mostwin's native Poland in the mid-1980s and trained mental health professionals to use the model in helping families of troubled youth. Later, after the dissolution of the Soviet Union in the 1990s, Mostwin was allowed back in her native country to train therapists along with Clark in the use of this model to families. The government of Poland in the early 1990s adopted the process as a way to help families transitioning from communist society to the emerging democracy of the time.

The use of a team approach to family intervention requires an initial output of therapist time and can be perceived by some as too costly to implement as an effective treatment model.

Mostwin (1980a, p. 215) addresses the concerns of critics who might think that applying so many people to one family as a costly extravagance, by comparing family mental health team professionals working in the way surgeons work on individuals as a team. Oftentimes multiproblem clients will have the involvement of many community professionals. Surgery usually requires several physicians in concert working on a patient. Mostwin encourages community agencies to come together in this treatment model. The dynamic action of the team working together in a short-term fashion is intended to save money for an organization. Whelley (1977) shares that her Catholic Charities agency in New York was able to compare the number of treatment hours for the STMFI model versus working with clients on an individual basis and found cost value. In this comparison of treatment hours, the agency spent 96 therapy hours using STMFI versus 216 therapy hours using a more individual model of treatment. Whelley's organization surmised that working in an intense dynamic team fashion with families has the potential to save time while providing effective treatment.

Despite the logic of short-term team therapy, this model has not been widely accepted and adopted by agencies across the United States. Many people were trained in the model but were unable to bring the process into full use in their after-training practice locations. After Ron Clark left his teaching position at Catholic University in Washington, DC, the Family Studies Center closed and students stopped being trained in the STMFI model at the university. Mostwin continued teaching the STMFI model in training centers at Loyola College, but the process did not have another teacher at that facility when Mostwin retired from the college in 1987. Before retiring, Mostwin promoted the STMFI process through conferences at Loyola College and changed the name of the process from the Short-Term Multidimensional Family Intervention model of practice to the Life Space Approach and then to Ecological Therapy (1982). The name changed because the concept of ecological practice better identified Mostwin's sense of addressing the family need by "promoting the mental health of the person in the family by exploring and building bridges with community resources" (Mostwin, 1982, p. iii).

BEYOND THE STMFI MODEL

While the STMFI or Ecological Model may have a lack of widespread use, the technique of the family life space drawing is a process that can be an enduring and useful technique used by counselors and therapists without the connection to the STMFI or Ecological Model of intervention. The FLSD owes its inspiration to the visual mapping of field theory to recognize personal and environmental influences affecting families. The FLSD is an expressive and task-centered projective technique that helps to identify family members and understand communication processes within the system, and it does not have to be applied within the confines of the STMFI model (Geddes & Medway, 1977). This technique can be used to discover family information by diminishing stress in the client and interactively learning about the biopsychosocial factors affecting the client. It also has the potential for clients to nonverbally disclose information.

This process can be used similarly in the way that the genogram process has been used by many therapists who do not follow the original treatment style of family systems therapy created by Murray Bowen. Therapists have adapted the genogram visual to other family treatment modalities (McGoldrick, Gerson, & Petry, 2008). The FLSD can be adapted to use with any type of mental health intervention, if only as a way to engage and learn about family psychosocial situations.

The many graduates and students of the trainings of the STMFI groups took the process of the FLSD and utilized it in their work settings, applying it to various professional counseling settings. The life space concept of the process can be applied to every family system orientation of intervention. Utilizing the FLSD in the first session can adapt to whatever theoretical approach a mental health professional might want to utilize. The FLSD can be completed with individuals, couples, and families. Clark and Beeton have adapted the process of the FLSD and used it to help organizations such as businesses and churches to identify systemic relationships within their groups.

Mostwin (1982, p. iii) informs in her last seminar monograph that her work embodies a "holistic view of the human situation" and that she still stresses the importance of a time-limited, dynamic creative therapy that helps to reconstruct and restructure a family situation. Mostwin (1982, p. iii) expands her philosophical beliefs that the use of "symbolic, nonverbal expression of feelings" will work with the "forces of nature" in the therapeutic process to support the family and the foundations of society.

SUMMARY

Danuta Mostwin created the FLSD as a way to engage and assess families participating in a treatment model designed to provide short-term treatment to troubled youth. The short-term treatment, also known as STMFI, focused on getting to know the family though the FLSD and then use the process as a starting point for designing interventions to help the family reorganize itself. The FLSD was used by many graduate students and community mental health providers. As a result of using this process both in internships and work settings, the process evolved and took on other applications other than following the STMFI model. Examining the motivations and original designs of Danuta Mostwin helps users to grasp the ideas of the visual representations of family members. The visual representations open the door toward helping individuals within a family context to share their story and eventually creating more functional ways of interacting in the family and, ultimately, society.

References

Banning, F. M., & Zinni, C. (1980). Alter-ego technique: A stimulus for communication. In D. Mostwin (Ed.), *Life space approach to the study and treatment of a family*. Washington, DC: The Catholic University of America.

Clark, R. (1980). Family life space in action. In D. Mostwin (Ed.), *Life space approach to the study and treatment of a family*. Washington, DC: The Catholic University of America.

Geddes, M., & Medway, J. (1977). The symbolic drawing of the family life space. *Family Process*, 16, 219–228.

Germain, C. (1973). An ecological perspective in casework practice. *Social Casework*, 54, 323–330.

Hartman, A. (2003). Comments on diagrammatic assessment of family relations. *Reflections summer*, 41–43.

Medway, J., & Geddes, M. (1976). The use of the alter-ego technique in short term multidimensional family intervention. In D. Mostwin (Ed.), *The social dimension of family treatment*. Washington, DC: The Catholic University of America.

McGoldrick, M., Gerson, R., & Petry, S. (2008). *Genograms: Assessment and intervention* (3rd ed.). New York, NY: W. W. Norton & Co.

Mostwin, D. (1972). In search of ethnic identity. *Social Casework*, 53, 306–316.

Mostwin, D. (1974a). The place of social casework in the field of family treatment. In D. Mostwin (Ed.), *Seminar on social casework in the field of family treatment*. Washington, DC: The Catholic University of America.

Mostwin, D. (1974b). Multidimensional model of working with the family. *Social Casework*, 55(4), 209–215.

Mostwin, D. (1976a). Social dimension of family treatment. In D. Mostwin (Ed.), *The social dimension of family treatment*. Washington, DC: The Catholic University of America.

Mostwin, D. (1976b). Social work intervention with families in crisis of change. *Social Thought*, 2, 81–99.

Mostwin, D. (1977a). Social work intervention with families in crisis of change. In D. Mostwin (Ed.), *The social dimension of treatment: The American family: Continuing impact of ethnicity*. Washington, DC: The Catholic University of America.

Mostwin, D. (1980a). *Social dimension of family treatment*. Washington, DC: National Association of Social Workers Inc.

Mostwin, D. (1980b). Life space approach to the study and treatment of a family. In D. Mostwin (Ed.), *Life space approach to the study and treatment of a family*. Washington, DC: The Catholic University of America.

Mostwin, D. (1982). Introduction. In D. Mostwin (Ed.), *Ecological therapy: The family life space approach*. Baltimore, MD: Loyola College.

Mostwin, D., Clark, R., Depenbrock, B., McKee, J., & Picado, S. (1977). Short term multidimensional intervention with families in crisis: Use of the therapeutic team. In D. Mostwin (Ed.), *The social dimension of treatment: The American family: Continuing impact of ethnicity*. Washington, DC: The Catholic University of America.

Preister, S. (1974). Systems theory: A conceptual base for family treatment. In D. Mostwin (Ed.), *Social casework in the field of family treatment*. Washington, DC: National Catholic School of Social Service.

Whelley, J. N. (1977). The development of a family treatment program in a voluntary agency. In *The social dimension of treatment: The American family: Continuing impact of ethnicity* (pp. 181–193). Washington, DC: National Catholic School of Social Service.

CHAPTER THREE
Family Life Space Drawing: Theories Behind the Family Life Space Process

Introduction

Usually concepts in psychology and mental health are derived from many theoretical sources, and the process of the FLSD is not unusual in that respect. The FLSD grew out of many influences, but the overriding foundational theory that inspired the concept of the FLSD is the ecological perspective of working with clients. Ecological perspectives will view the client more in terms of an integrated system versus as an individual having intrapsychic stress and working out mental health issues from an individual basis. Focusing on the interactions of the clients with their ecosystem provides a life model based on strengths versus pathology (Germain, 1973). The client's ecosystem includes people they interact with, places, organizations, values, and other related information The ecological model recognizes that human development takes place in a "complex, reciprocal interaction between humans and all the people, objects, and symbols in the immediate environment" (Bronfenbrenner, 1994, p. 38). These environments will include many layers for people within themselves and their biology and time in history, as well as environmental systems within the family and their communities and the planet at large. The process of the FLSD has the potential to review all the various systems that might be influencing family members within any life space.

Social work has a long history of working with clients in their environment, and it is likely that Mostwin's social work education was a strong influence on her way to developing a systemic, ecological intervention. Working with families in the 1950s became an exciting treatment method that originated out of frustrations with the gaps in traditional psychoanalytic modes of treatment more common in that time frame (Bowen, 1976). Mostwin, like many mental health professionals of her time, was drawn to ecological concepts that involved treating families within the context of their internal and external environments. Mostwin gives credit to George Herbert Mead, Andras Anyal, Pierre Teilhard de Chardin, and Margaret Mead as strong philosophical and practical influences in her development as a family therapist (Mostwin, 1980a). Other systemic thinkers included Ludwig von Bertalanffy and Kurt Lewin. Our discussion will review some of the theories and techniques that served as inspiration for developing the FLSD along with connecting the theories to the application of the FLSD.

Systems Theory

The underlying theory that supports the concept of the FLSD is the influence of general systems theory. Ludwig von Bertalanffy, a biologist, offered his insights on the theory of the open system to the behavioral and social sciences (Bertalanffy, 1975, p. 32). These insights, which might be more commonly accepted now than at the time of their introduction in the late 1920s and the 1930s, offered that investigating a single part of an organism does not adequately provide a complete explanation of that organism (Bertalanffy, 1975, p. 152). General systems theory suggests a view that for true understanding of an organism one must see not only the elements of the system but also the interplay of those elements with each other within the environments they exist. Bertalanffy (1975, p. 157) describes general systems theory as an exploration of the whole. He further describes a system as a "set of elements standing in interrelation among themselves and with the environment" (Bertalanffy, 1975, p. 159). A system is described by Berrien (1968, p. vi) not only as components that interact with other but also as processing a boundary that filters inputs and outputs. It is a natural connection for family therapists to see systems theory as a conceptualization of approaching mental health treatment through the whole of the client's environment versus an individual focus.

Steven Preister (1974) organized systems concepts and characteristics as they applied to family therapy that used the FLSD in this way:

1. Systems are open or closed
2. Systems have boundaries
3. There are inputs and outputs to the system
4. Feedback is the way that systems regulate response to inputs and outputs
5. Homeostasis is the function of the system to find stability
6. Systems have functions of negative entropy that store information for future use
7. Differentiation is the process whereby a system grows and adapts
8. Equifinality is the concept that a final state can be obtained by various pathways.

These concepts are in line with general systems theory, which recognizes that living organisms are open and operate in response or the offering of a stimuli (Bertalanffy, 1975, p. 209).

Bowen (1976, p. 408) draws from general system theory by noting subsystems exist within the family as a whole. Subsystems exist in myriad possibilities. The first one starts with the individual, who is a member of the larger group, of the family. These subsystems can be parental, sibling, and any other variation within the family. Subsystems grow beyond the family to the community, society, and environment (suprasystems). When in therapy, these systems extend to therapists and all operate from inputs, outputs, and feedback loops. In the case of a family, each member is influencing all other members of the family back and forth all at the same time. Bowen (1976, p. 409) suggests that therapists become systems analysts in order to understand the interface of family problems and how perception and feedback affect family functioning.

The FLSD is a helpful process that operates from systemic perspectives by attempting to understand clients as part of a whole system. The FLSD will help to understand the family by identifying component parts of the system and defining subsystems within the system. The

FLSD will identify boundaries within the system and begin to explore how each member interacts and experiences other family members. The process will identify and begin to explore family and individual connections with outside organizations. Internal stresses that might be affecting individuals will be identified and visually presented. Through the interactive process of the FLSD, clients and therapist will have an opportunity to explore inputs and outputs that affect the system. The interactive process can provide clues as to how the family maintains homeostatic functions and how to begin reorganizing in ways that might become more functional in the future.

Ivan Boszormenyi-Nagy (1973) influenced the development of the FLSD by encouraging the recognition of multigenerational accounts of family justice and the legacy of family history, even if the issue is not immediately presenting itself in the session. Family ties and history influence present functioning. The FLSD reviews multigenerational family members even if they are not present in the session or have passed away.

General systems theory influences family therapy by expanding the client assessment in terms of its whole versus individual parts. The therapy focuses on the interactions within the subsystems, which are considered ecological living organisms that have multiple capacity for finding homeostatic functions (Nichols & Davis, 2017).

The FLSD is influenced by the emerging adaptations of general systems theory to family therapy. Several assumptions of operating in family therapy are assumed in the process. Nichols and Davis (2017, pp. 60–66) summarizes the following as working concepts of family therapy:

   Interpersonal context

   Circular causality

   Focus on process over content

   Family structure awareness

   Family life cycle considerations

   Gender and culture as focus of attention and concern.

The process of the FLSD identifies these concepts through the interactive process by defining family structure, exploring interpersonal connections, and reflecting on the experiences of one member over another in each specific situation.

Field Theory

Kurt Lewin was a German scientist who created field theory as an attempt to understand conceptualization of electromagnetic forces. Relating field theory to psychology was not an attempt to connect psychological dynamics to physical processes. The interplay of field theory and psychology was more of an attempt to analyze causal relationships and build scientific constructs (Lewin, 1943, 1951, pp. 43–59). Lewin's work was groundbreaking in its day because he was one of the first theorists to offer the idea that environment contributed to personality development and behavior.

Lewin graphically describes the concept of life space as:

> In summary, one can say that behavior and development depend upon the state of the person (P) and his environment (E) have to be viewed as variables which are

mutually dependent upon each other. In other words, to understand or to predict behavior, the person and his environment have to be considered as one constellation of interdependent factors. We call the totality of these factors the life space (LSp) of that individual, and write $B = F(P, E) = F(LSp)$. The life space, therefore, includes both the person and his psychological environment.

(Lewin, 1951, 239–240)

Behavior can be determined by many co-existing facts that take into account the person and his environment (Lewin, 1938). His use of hodological (recognition of pathways) space shows closeness or distance; it can mirror biological facts, represent social problems, and put cognitive facts together with dynamical facts (p. 3). Lewin graphically represented behaviors and conflict and represented these constructs with images that involved circles and oblong shapes with letters that represented forces.

Figure 3.1 gives an idea of how Lewin would see the progression of influence on the person.

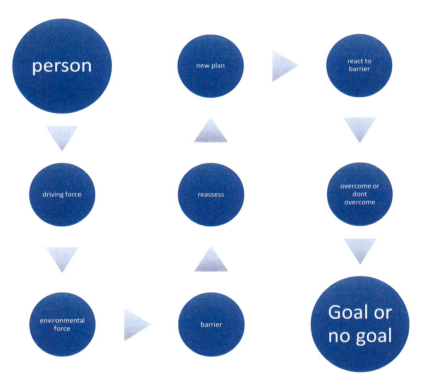

Figure 3.1 This illustration shows causal pathways that describe how the person starts with driving forces-that affect environmental forces, with potential barriers that arise and the person reassesses, develops a new plan and subsequently reacts to a new barrier that they overcome or not thus achieving or not achieving a goal. Lewin would also suggest that the forces go both ways and between the forces in constant feedback loops.

Lewin (1951, p. 57) thought that psychologists would be interested in understanding people in the here and now by focusing on the following areas:

1. The life space, which includes the person and their psychological environment, focusing on anxieties, tensions, goals, motivations, and ideals among other psychological factors;
2. Many processes in the physical and social world that might not be immediately affecting the individual at that time;
3. Boundary zones: the perceptions of family members for outside and inside forces.

Lewin (1951, pp. 4, 29) believed that mathematical formulations could be applied to psychological interactions within the life space. He recognized that measurement was in the early stages, but he did not hesitate to graphically depict life space interactions.

Field theory mathematicians could develop future processes for effectively measuring family interactions.

Mostwin (1980a, pp. 9–10) adapted the concept of the life space and applied the visual interactive spatial drawing as part of family assessment for her treatment model. her way of using Lewin's life space concept in this way:

$$LS = P + E$$

Or, life space equals the person and the environment.

Mostwin further indicates that behavior is a function of the person's environment. So, for Mostwin, the family life space equals the family and the environment and that family mental health is reflected in the family life space.

The formula for the View of the family life space is illustrated:

$$B = f(L) = f(P, E)$$

where B = behavior, f = function, L = life, P = person, and E = environment. Behavior is the function of a person's life space and subsequently a function of the person and their environment (Mostwin, 1980a).

Mostwin adapted Lewin's theories to understand clients within the confines of their environment at a specific moment. The FLSD operates with the assumption that people occupy space that is related to other people and organizations within their environment. Mostwin (1980b p. 4) draws from Lewin by seeing behavior as goal oriented and that life space representations can be influenced by connections to people and objects. These representations will not be static and can change with goals being accomplished or not completed. Graphic representation can show barriers to accomplishing goals. Knowing the family life space allows for more than just obtaining facts from clients; it represents the interplay of the facts and how these unique configurations might be determining the specific behavior of family members (Lewin, 1951, p. 238).

The FLSD technique allows clients to report on information about individuals that make up their life space, both living and deceased. The FLSD process includes psychological factors and environmental or institutional factors. The act of completing the drawing provides a symbolic visual representation of the client's life space (Mostwin, 1980a). The FLSD provides the client and therapist with an orientation toward the whole of the person and allows for a possibility of revealing subconscious information (Mostwin, 1977). Field theory stresses the importance of recognizing the whole field (Lewin, 1951). The graphic representation of the FLDS provides an illustration of the client's life space concerning people, institutional factors, and life stresses. The graphic symbolic representation recognizes that each of the symbols is interactively influencing each other in a back-and-forth fashion. It would be next to impossible to truly work effectively with a family system without recognition of all of these factors. Fortunately, the visual aspects of the FLSD provide a picture that helps client and therapist to identify areas of concern that will define the formulations of the treatment plan.

COMMUNICATION THEORY

Communication theory in the practice of family therapy emerged after observing communication patterns between schizophrenic populations and their families. The research project was started by Gregory Bateson and involved Jay Haley, John Weakland, William Fry Jr., and Don Jackson. What emerged after this research was the recognition that the interventions that apply for improving communication among schizophrenic families could apply to nonpsychotic people as well. The research group focused on the concept of cybernetic function of behavior. Feedback loops provide a reinforcement to any type of behavior, whether it be labeled positive or negative (Weakland, 1976). Communication theory focuses on interactional aspects of the behavior versus exploring underlying issues that affect the problem. Communication theorists will examine the situation as a problem that gets reinforced and produces a functional or nonfunctional experience in the family system. The focus is on the here and now situation and ways that it is currently affecting the problem brought into therapy. Communication patterns are observed and identified with the notation that incongruent messages often create distress and symptoms that create problems in a system (Weakland, 1976, p. 119)

Becvar and Becvar (2013, p. 70) recognized that communication theorists offer that communication is both a verbal and nonverbal process, and that on some levels nonverbal communications are able to convey more meaning than words, especially if words are incongruent with the message. The FLSD attempts to obtain communication from the family on both the verbal and nonverbal levels through the symbolic placements of the drawing. The family drawing process is able to explore incongruences by noting placements and communications lines and discussing the subjective meanings of each with family members.

The FLSD focuses on the here and now and is also exploring feedback loops that may help dysfunctional patterns to continue. It also helps to define the possibility of new emerging patterns that will create more functional behavior within the system. The drawing facilitates clarification of communicated messages by illustrating visual representations of incongruences. The interactive process of completing the FLSD recognizes that the message symbolically represented by the client is not just in the meaning of the words but also how the words affect behavior. An example might be that a family member would state that they are close to another family member, but the drawing might illustrate a different picture. This is a situation where it is good to explore the visual representation with the verbal message.

Cybernetic communication patterns observe family rules, negative feedback loops, sequences of interaction, and what happens when the systems-accustomed feedback is ineffective in triggering a positive feedback loop (Nichols & Davis, 2017). The process of exploring the family life space recognizes these communication components and looks for information concerning the possible connection of these operations in the evolving FLSD process.

The symbolic representations of the symbols in the drawing also provide another level of information, as the facilitator/therapists can seek to discover the meaning for the client that they applied to the placement and size of the symbol. Recognizing the individual specific meanings that family members apply to the placement of symbols in the FLSD is compatible with emerging social constructivist theories in family therapy. In postmodern applications of family interventions, therapists are operating not so much as an expert but as a facilitator (Becvar & Becvar, 2013). Current therapists can operate in a similar fashion by not being the interpreter of symbolic meaning and expect that the clients will form their own meanings in the FLSD graphic display

EXPRESSIVE THERAPY TECHNIQUES

As the field of family therapy developed, many innovative and creative therapies originated to treat family problems (Goldenberg & Goldenberg, 1996). The FLSD has a similarity to some of the expressive therapies developing at the time (Nichols & Davis, 2017, pp. 138–139). Some of these include family sculpting, family art, and the use of puppets. All of these expressive techniques involve the use of some tools other than verbal communication.

The family sculpting technique provides an expressive tool and allows clients to physically place family members in relation to each other (Duhl, Kantor, & Duhl, 1973). The family sculpting process asks clients to physically demonstrate relationships within a family. The family sculpting process is a way of illustrating the family life space. The experiential process also provides an experiential process to nonverbally, symbolically represent family relationship patterns. Family puppets use the puppets to represent family interactions.

Art therapy moved from individual focus on individual drawings and developed treatments oriented to families recognizing that graphic instruments facilitate communication between family members. Art therapy with families can provide an expressive activity which the family can complete simultaneously all together providing indirect means of communication (Kwiatkowska, 1967, p. 1). In addition, the act of creating art together as a family can lessen superego effects and provide symbolic unconscious images of feelings. Family art therapy allows families to work together and potentially provide projective material about the family and themselves in their artwork through this expressive tool. Bing (1970) demonstrated in her research of family art that family drawings can have a diagnostic, therapeutic, and research benefit. Family drawing research indicates that family art can portray information about family organization, structure, as well as demonstrating information about other relevant dimensions about the content of the family situation, projective information related to the size of the drawing, and issues related to isolation of family members. Gennari and Tamanza (2013) are developing coding systems as a way to measure variables related to emotional, interactive, and relational aspects of the family drawing. These coding procedures address the need for research of the graphical aspects of the FLSD.

Dr. Mostwin worked with many art therapists during the 1970's and incorporated art therapy into her Short-Term Multidimensional Intervention with families (Hertzberg & Geddes, 1976). Kwiatkowska's work in art therapy influenced the development of the FLSD as Mostwin and Kwiatkowska often consulted with each other as colleagues (Mostwin, 1977).

The FLSD is an expressive task oriented tool, much like the tools of family art therapy. The family is asked to symbolically draw their family's life space on the same page and in a similar time frame, expressing unconscious indirect messages in a nonthreatening manner.

The FLSD makes use of simple and basic images to help the client to reveal the inner and outer world (Mostwin, 1980b).

Other Theoretical Influences

Role theory and crisis theory have been noted by students who studied the results of using the STMFI model (Allman and Madigan, 1974; Dailey, 1980). These theories are not necessary to utilize in the adaptations of using the FLSD. Role theory speaks to recognition of guidelines for social interaction. Role theory identifies that role complementarity leads to harmonious connections and disequilibrium if the opposite occurs (Spiegel, 1971). The FLSD has the potential to identify roles and the way they interface among family members. The interactive process of completing the drawing presents opportunity for attention to these details.

Crisis theory addresses the dynamic forces that looks to enter the system when the system is in crisis to help facilitate immediate change. The short-term nature of the STMFI model is dependent on the crisis concept so that the family will be mobilized and enact emergent processes that would set into effect the positive aspects of systemic regrouping. Crisis theory research indicates that people are less defensive and possibly open to change when in current crisis states (Halpern, 1973).

Symbolic Interactionism

The FLSD concept developed with some influence of George Herbert Mead (1934) and the subsequent emerging sociological concepts of symbolic interactionism. Mostwin's theory of the family life space and its focus on ecological concepts is congruent with the sociological concepts of symbolic interactionism, which notes that we develop the concept of the self through interactions with others (Billson, 1994). Symbolic interactionism recognizes that symbols represent abstract things and can be words or objects and gestures (Redmond, 2015).

Human communication takes place through symbolic interactions that include nonverbal gestures, and significant images which include agreed-upon conventional symbols that have the same meaning for all (DeFleur, D'Antonio, & DeFleur, 1972).

Collins (1982) reviewed family therapy interventions for evidence of symbolic interaction theory and discovered that most models of family therapy apply some element of symbolic theory in their practice and theory. Collins included Mostwin's ecological life space theory in the review and observed that Mostwin's approach had implicit and explicit use of the symbolic theory. The FLSD provides an example of using symbols in the drawing to represent self and relationships with others, drawing from the clients' own experience as an explicit manifestation. The implicit application of symbolic theory is manifested when therapists use information obtained from clients and then provide interactions with each other as alter ego family members.

Redmond (2015) defines the guiding principles of symbolic interactionism through four points:

1. Our behavior is based on meanings we develop
2. The meanings we create derive from our social interactions
3. We apply an interpretive process within ourselves
4. The self continues to adapt and make new meanings through these interactions.

Mostwin would most likely offer that the visual placements of the clients completing the FLSD will represent their interactional experiences with family members in the content of the drawing. The drawing has the potential to utilize the innate process of symbolically expressing and experiencing others in everyday life. Because life space elements have the potential for new adaptations, changes will be noticed if effective interventions have been introduced in the therapy process. These changes have been noted by Mostwin and others in reviewing the FLSD of clients as they start therapy and after they have completed the therapy process (Dailey, 1980; Mostwin, 1982). The FLSD is just another representational opportunity for communication among human beings. The symbols in the FLSD have the potential to illustrate the sense of self that others derive from their interactions with others in the family and community environment.

SUMMARY

The FLSD has a rich conceptual heritage that draws from many theories but operates foundationally from systemic, ecological, and symbolic interactionism. Mostwin was heavily influenced by systemic thinking and recognized that the environmental factors, as emphasized by Lewin, played an important role in developing the life space of not just individuals but families all together. Communication theory helped to influence the way Mostwin interpreted information gained from the FLSD by expanding communication processes beyond just verbal representations. The main focus of the FLSD process creates an experiential, expressive opportunity for people to represent themselves and family relationships. Symbolic representations have the potential to communicate on nonverbal levels and the FLSD creates a visual image to investigate communications with family members starting on a nonverbal level. The various theories that support the development of the FLSD process provide light and interesting possibilities on what the meaning of the symbols might reveal. These possibilities have to do with potential information about self-esteem, experience of others, and environmental factors within the life space. The drawing illustrates the life space of the family by illustrating with symbols that include not just the individuals in the family but also symbols for environmental factors, along with symbols for psychological stressors affecting individuals internally and externally.

REFERENCES

Allman, M. A., & Madigan, M. P. (1974). Presentation of some research findings from master's thesis. In D. Mostwin (Ed.), *Social casework in the field of family treatment*. Washington DC: The Catholic University of America.
Becvar, D. S., & Becvar, R. J. (2013). *Family therapy: A systemic integration* (8th ed.). Upper Saddle River, NJ: Pearson.
Berrien, K. (1968). *General and social systems*. New Brunswick, NJ: Rutgers University Press.
Bertalanffy, L. (1975). *Perspectives on general systems theory: Scientific and philosophical studies*. New York, NY: George Braziller.
Billson, J. M. (1994). Society and self: A symbolic interactionist framework for sociological Practice. *Clinical Sociology Review*, 12(1). Retrieved from http://digitalcommons.wayne.edu/csr?vol12/iss1/11
Bing, E. (1970). The conjoint family drawing. *Family Process*, 9, 173–194.
Boszormenyi-Nagy, I., & Spark, G. (1973). *Invisible loyalties: Reciprocity in intergenerational family therapy*. Hagerstown, MD: Harper & Row Publishers.
Bowen, M. (1976). Theory in the practice of psychotherapy. In P. Guerin (Ed.), *Family therapy: theory and practice*. New York, NY: Gardner Press Inc.

Bronfenbrenner, U. (1994). Ecological models of human development. In *International encyclopedia of education* (vol. 3, 2nd ed.). Oxford: Elsevier.

Collins, W. A. (1982). Implementation of symbolic interaction in the theory and practice of family therapy. In D. Mostwin (Ed.), *Ecological therapy: The family life space approach*. Baltimore, MD: Loyola College.

Dailey, K. (1980). The use of the life space drawing in treatment. In D. Mostwin (Ed.), *Life space approach to the study of family treatment*. Washington, DC: The Catholic University of America.

DeFleur, M. L., D'Antonio, W. V., & DeFleur, L. B. (1972). *Sociology: Man and society*. Glenview, IL: Scott, Foresman & Co.

Duhl, F. J., Kantor, D., & Duhl, B. S. (1973). Learning space and action in family therapy. A primer of sculpture. In D. A. Bloch (Ed.), *Techniques of family psychotherapy: A primer*. New York, NY: Grune & Stratton.

Gennari, M., & Tamanza, G. (2013). Conjoint family drawing: A technique for family clinical assessment. *Procedia: Social and Behavioral Sciences*, 113, 91–10.

Germain, C. B. (1973). An ecological perspective in casework practice. *Social Casework*, 54, 323–330.

Goldenberg, I., & Goldenberg, H. (1996). *Family therapy: An overview* (4th ed.). Pacific Grove, CA: Brooks/Cole Publishing Co.

Halpern, H. A. (1973). Crisis theory: A definitional study. *Community Mental Health Journal*, 9(4), 342–349.

Hertzberg, C., & Geddes, M. (1976). Art therapy with siblings: A dimension of family treatment. In D. Mostwin (Ed.), *The social dimension of family treatment*. Washington, DC: The Catholic University of America.

Kwiatkowska, H. A. (1967). Family art therapy. *Family Process*, 6, 37–55.

Lewin, K. (1938, 2013). *The conceptual representation and the measurement of psychological forces*. Mansfield Centre, CT: Martino Publishing.

Lewin, K. (1943). Defining the field at a given time. *Psychological Review*, 50, 292–310.

Lewin, K. (1951). *Field theory in social sciences: Selected theoretical papers*. New York, NY: Harper & Row.

Mead, G. H. (1934). *Mind, self and society*. Chicago, IL: University of Chicago Press.

Mostwin, D. (1977). Social work intervention with families in crisis of change. In D. Mostwin (Ed.), *The social dimension of treatment: The American family: Continuing impact of ethnicity*. Washington, DC: The Catholic University of America.

Mostwin, D. (1980a). *Social dimension of family treatment*. Washington, DC: National Association of Social Workers Inc.

Mostwin, D. (1980b). Life space approach to the study and treatment of a family. In D. Mostwin (Ed.), *Life space approach to the study and treatment of a family*. Washington, DC: The Catholic University of America.

Mostwin, D. (1982). Predelinquent youth and their families. In D. Mostwin (Ed.), *Ecological therapy: The family life space approach*. Baltimore, MD: Loyola College.

Nichols, M., & Davis, S. (2017). *Family therapy: concepts and methods* (11th ed.). Boston, MA: Pearson.

Preister, S. (1974). Systems theory: A conceptual base for family treatment. In D. Mostwin (Ed.), *Social casework in the field of family treatment*. Washington, DC: The Catholic University of America.

Redmond, M. V. (2015). Symbolic interactionism. *English Technical Reports and White Papers*, 4. Retrieved from http://lib.dr.iastate.edu/engl_reports/4

Spiegel, J. (1971). *Transaction: The interplay between individual, family and society*. New York, NY: Science House, Inc.

Weakland, J. (1976). Communication theory and clinical change. In P. Guerin (Ed.), *Family therapy: Theory and practice*. New York, NY: Gardner Press, Inc.

CHAPTER FOUR
Family Life Space Drawing: Ten Steps to Complete the Family Life Space Drawing

Symbolic Representation

Ancient people used symbols to express spirituality and to apply meaning to life. One of the symbols used since ancient times is the mandala defined as a circular figure that represents the universe in Hindu and Buddhist symbolism (Oxford English Dictionary, 2018). The symbol of the circle becomes the starting point for creating the FLSD. This ancient symbol helps to create a representation that will not only allow for the flow of the client identifying information but also create an opportunity for tapping into something that has the potential to facilitate emerging unconscious information.

In his book, *Man and His Symbols,* Carl Jung (1968, p. 230) references the importance of the circle as an image that provides a symbol of order and a symbolic representation of the human psyche. The circle can also symbolically represent the inner being and serve as a focal point for meditation and a vehicle to bring inner peace. Jung noticed that the image of the circle appeared in the dreams of people with religious and nonreligious backgrounds. He connects these images to an intent to find wholeness and inner peace. Jung also sees the representations of the images of the square and circle as an intent to bring basic life factors into consciousness.

Mostwin (1980a, p. 61) references these concepts by offering that the focus on drawing the first symbol of the large circle helps family members to relieve tension and tap into unconscious thoughts when first engaging in the therapeutic process. Mostwin (1982) recognizes the potentially meditative component of using the mandala symbol as something that helps to tap into unconscious concentration and a sense of order. Geddes and Medway (1977, p. 227) observed that in their experience, the process of completing the FLSD is effective for lowering anxiety and reducing blocks to engaging in the first diagnostic encounter. They offer that the task is simple and allows people to engage in the therapeutic process before the more difficult aspects of therapy occur. The symbolic nonverbal representation is an important component of this process.

Ten Steps to Complete the FLSD Process

Materials needed:

A. An easel with a large white flip chart of paper to complete the drawing, especially if completing the process with more than one person. Some have used a blackboard or whiteboard. If using something that cannot be saved, such as a whiteboard or blackboard, please be sure to save the image by taking a picture or making a paper copy for your own records. It is possible to use large newsprint paper taped to the wall. The best way to complete a FLSD is to have a large blank space available in order to create the drawing that will allow all family members to see the paper while it is in the process of completion. A regular sheet of copy paper can be used if completing the drawing with one person.

B. Colored markers or colored chalk for use with a blackboard. Each family member needs to have a different color to symbolically represent themselves.

C. A blank sheet of paper for the facilitator and a pencil or marker to make notes on the drawing.

Step One: Introducing the Process

New clients are greeted and asked to complete a process that will help the therapist and client in getting to know each other and will help to share more information about the family. Sometimes the concept of using symbols to represent brands or ideas is referenced to the client. An example of such introductory remarks might be:

> We all know that symbols are used to represent things in our society. An example of this might be the American flag. It is a symbol of the United States but not a real picture of the United States. We are going to develop something like that today, we are going to symbolically represent your family by using simple geometric shapes that will allow us get to know each other better.

It is important to reassure people that this effort will not require any special artistic ability and that there are no right or wrong answers. The therapist then allows the people present to pick out separate colors to enable them to represent themselves. Sometimes the therapist will hand a marker to participants, especially if some resistance to the process might be apparent.

Step Two: The Facilitator Draws the First Symbol

The facilitator will then draw attention to the whiteboard and sometimes smooth the paper. It is important that all family members are focused on the white sheet. It might even be necessary to call attention to the board if someone is distracted. The facilitator then slowly draws a large circle on the board while saying:

> This symbol represents your family. The symbol represents the family you created together and the family you came from. It is your present and your past and some hints to the future. The circle is then reemphasized by circling it with the facilitator's hand and again stating that this symbol represents your family. This process of circling the circle with the facilitator's hand can take place two or three times.

Please note that the facilitator references the word "symbol" and does not call the drawing a circle. All of these actions are designed to help the clients to access meditative components.

Step Three: Family Members Each Draw a Personal Symbol

Family members are then again focused on the large sheet and told by the facilitator while circling the first symbol: "if this symbol represents your family and you use a similar symbol like this [at that time the facilitator takes another piece of paper and draws a smaller circle on a piece of paper, as an example] represents you, where would you be or where would you see yourself?"

Once again, a family member is encouraged to come to the board and retold: "if this symbol (pointing to the larger circle) represents your family and this symbol pointing to the circle on the outside paper represents you, where would you be?" Oftentimes people will ask, "In the circle"? The facilitators best response is "anywhere you see yourself is the right answer." People often need reassurance that whatever they come up with is the correct answer and acceptable. It is useful to remind people that they are to place themselves where they presently see themselves versus where they would like to be or think they ought to be placed in the drawing. Sometimes they will act puzzled and be confused with the process. Clients need encouragement to just go with their first thought. The facilitator needs to keep saying the instructions over a few times if necessary: "if this symbol (pointing on the large board) represents your family and this symbol (pointing to the image on the small paper) represents you . . . where would you be?" Or the facilitator could ask, "where do you see yourself?"

If the client is hesitant or wonders where they are supposed to place themselves, it is important to be reassuring and encouraging that it will all be good no matter what they do. We often say everything is a right answer.

Clients then get out of their seats and one by one come to the board and place themselves using the symbol in their color where they see themselves in relation to the larger family symbol. We do not provide direction on placement either in or out of the circle. We prefer to allow the client to have a blank slate of direction to enable unconscious processes to have full manifestation. This is a departure from early forms of this process referenced in Geddes and Medway (1977, p. 221), where people were encouraged to place themselves inside the circle. Each person in the room is asked to place themselves on the drawing. In the case of a family with an identified family member as the stated reason for coming to counseling, we usually do not start with that family member. We ask a sibling or another family member to go first. This allows the family to begin the process of seeing family problems as a systemic situation versus an individually based problem that needs fixing.

Step Four: Placement of Significant People

After the last family member, or spouse if it is a couple, has placed themselves on the drawing, they are then asked to draw symbols for other family members who are not in the room. In the case of a couple completing the drawing, the last partner will then be asked to show symbols for children who are not present. Clients are asked to place other family members on the drawing such as parents, grandparents, siblings, and in-laws. Clients are encouraged to include deceased family members even if they did not have a living personal relationship. It is important to include ex-spouses or partners, especially if the previous relationship included children.

Every time a symbol is placed on the drawing, it is good to recap the placement by saying something like "You see yourself in that part, is that right?" Or "you see your children here?" This is an opportunity to begin talking about the client's personal information: "Tell me about your children? How old are they? Do they live with you, and if not, where do they live?" Oftentimes a client will begin to draw in significant people, but it is good to slow things down by asking about the people they are symbolically representing. An example might be in asking about the adult's family of origin: "Where do you see your parents?" After the client places them on the drawing, the facilitator asks about the parents, such as "are your parents living? Do they live together?" These questions are launching pads to learn about family history and experiences in close relationships. We ask about siblings and birth order and extended family members related to siblings, such as in-laws and nieces and nephews. We can learn about children from previous relationships and connections to the parents of those children. We encourage people to identify placements for all people, including past relationships and miscarriages or other deceased family members.

Clients who have a history of being adopted are asked to place biological parents on the life space as well as adoptive parents. We encourage this process even if the person was adopted at birth and never had a relationship with the biological parent. Completing this process in this way allows for an opportunity to learn about the client's background and receive insight as to unspoken issues.

Completing the drawing with multiple family members allows for obtaining a perspective on how different family members might experience the same person. In a family, one person might see the grandmother in an entirely different placement than another family member. Couples who are completing the drawing as part of couples counseling will both draw the children symbolically from their perspective. Once again, each member of the couple might see the children in a different place. Clients are informed that even though they share a life space they might have a different perspective on placement of other people affecting the life space. This is a great opportunity to start initiating the concept of individuation of family members especially if another family member wants to encourage someone to place a person in one spot. Facilitators need to encourage the individual response and support that concept. While making the point for individuation of family members, we do note that sometimes people will see family members in the same place and circle that spot with their color to signify agreement.

After all family members, current and past are included, we ask about family pets and let each person include family pets wherever they see them in the life space. The placement of family pets has an opportunity to provide insight into the life of individual family members (Barker, Barker, Dawson, & Knisely, 1997). Past evaluations of the FLSD often revealed that pets can be found in emotionally significant places in the family life space (Mostwin, 1980a).

Finally, each person is asked if there is anyone else who is like family to them. This is opportunity to learn about other important people who play a role in the family's life. People will sometimes place friends or other important people (like Alcoholics Anonymous sponsors) as part of the FLSD. All symbolic placements provide a catalyst for learning about the family and individual members.

During the process of placing significant others and pets, the facilitator has an opportunity to engage in the joining process by finding ways to connect with the client. If the client indicates they have brothers and the therapist is comfortable with sharing personal information, they can say things such as "I have brothers too" or "I was the youngest in my family too, I know what that is like" if it facilitates connecting with the client. Other ways to connect with the client can be facilitated by making validating statements connected to the client's situation, such as "it must be fun to have traveled so much" or "that it is a challenge when parents are reported to have died young from difficult circumstances." All client information is an opportunity to make a human connection and let the client know that you are interested in their life story.

Step Five: Environmental or Institutional Factors

After all of the people and pets related to the life space are presented by each family member, the last one completing their placements is then introduced to the next symbol.

The clients are asked to represent influences that affect the family, but which are not people, by using this symbol (and a symbol of the square is drawn on the extra sheet of paper to demonstrate the symbol). Once again, we do not use the word "square" or indicate if it is small or large. By limiting the instructions and making them vague, it allows clients to make their own projective representations, which we can ask about later after the FLSD is completed. The symbol is also defined in ways that the client can understand, and clients are informed that it can be an institutional or environmental involvement.

The clients receive instruction that the new symbol represents the person's sense of institutions such as jobs, school, clubs, hobbies, associations, spiritual organizations, and any activity or place that influences time and energy. Institutional factors can also include community agencies such as courts, hospitals, and public organizations. Once again, the clients receive instruction to consider their first thought in making placement. Clients also receive encouragement that each answer is acceptable. Each person in the client group takes a turn using their own specific colored marker. Each person may include the same institutional factor identifying their own unique perspective on the placement of that factor. An example might include different perspectives on the placement of spiritual institutions and work. During the course of taking time to make the placements for institutional factors, the therapist is able to learn more information about the client and each family member's perspective of the same institution. As is often the case, people in the same life space do not have the same experience of an institutional factor. The visual expression of the FLSD often reveals that concept without anyone saying a word about the differences.

The therapist notices the placements and environmental symbols, and asks questions and begins to join the family system (Mostwin, 1980b). The therapist/counselor with each placement or indication of an environmental factor can ask questions about the activity and sometimes make comments about the symbol, especially if it is significantly large or small, such as "it looks like you have a lot of activities and involvements affecting you; does it ever get overwhelming?" Or the facilitator can offer a statement that is validating or affirming about the activity, either in an appropriate positive or concerned way. These types of interactions create client and therapist connections that facilitate the development of the therapeutic relationship.

The environmental factors symbol provides an expanded amount of information about the family life space. Geddes and Medway (1977) note that the process of including environmental factors is something that is important for biopsychosocial assessment and has not often been seen in expressive tools and techniques. Hartman (1978) advanced the pictorial concept of including environmental factors in family evaluations with the development of the ecomap by providing opportunities for identifying environmental factors affecting families. The ecomap is often mentioned as a qualitative assessment tool in books and articles about family assessment (Ghanbaripanah & Mustaffa, 2012; Thomlison, 2016). Mostwin takes the concept of identifying environmental factors to an expanded dimension by providing a projective opportunity through the process of the FLSD. Clients not only identify environmental factors but they also give insight as to the influence and impact of these factors on family life. Once again, the facilitator does not provide direction on where to place these institutional factors. The facilitator remains neutral and does not provide instructions as to whether or not these factors would be placed in or out of the main circle of the life space.

In the early development of the FLSD, Mostwin (1974) designed the process in a more guided and structured manner by asking clients to place people inside the circle and environmental factors outside the circle. As time went on and the process was being used with more families, it was decided to eliminate any direction concerning placement and allow clients to place the symbols wherever they preferred to place them (Mostwin, Clark, Depenbrock, McKee, & Picado, 1977).

Step Six: Identifying Stress Factors

After placing the symbols representing the environmental factors for each person in the room completing the drawing, the facilitator introduces the next symbol. The facilitator might say something like:

> Our next symbol for this process represents stress that affects you and family. Stress is often considered something negative in our life, but stress can also be connected to something positive. I can say that for me, it is stressful to raise children, but it is a stress I am grateful to have. Using this symbol to represent stress (drawing the shape of a triangle on the separate sheet of white paper), please let me know where you see your stressors.

Sometimes it is important to identify the concept of stress in words that can be understood by the client. Sometimes children will not relate to the word stress, so it is important to ask the client if they understand what is meant by the word stress. Another word we use for stress is a worry or concern that one might have.

Each family member has a chance to identify current stresses that face the individual or the family. By identifying the stressors and locating them, with their own colored marker, in relation to the life space, clients are able to offer statements related to what is happening in their life. They are also able to begin the conversation with the therapist about their reason for seeking counseling support in the first place. It is important to note that the process of placing symbols in this drawing allows the therapist to make comments that facilitate the joining process. Therapists can find ways to relate or offer a validating comment connected to the identified stressors that will facilitate the development of the therapeutic relationship.

Step Seven: Optional Symbols – Number One Concern, Greatest Frustration

Ron Clark added two symbols to the FLSD that might be potential expansions to the concept of the stress symbols (Clark & Beeton, 2000). These symbols continue the conversation of getting to know the family system by asking about issues related to the client's deepest concerns and frustrations. These symbols are optional and may be used if more information is needed and time allows.

After each family member completes the stress symbol, the last person at the drawing board receives the request to consider their number one concern and represent it in the drawing by using the symbol of a question mark. The symbol is also illustrated for the clients on a separate sheet of paper. Each family member is asked to place their symbol in relation to the FLSD.

After placing the symbol related to the number one concern, the facilitator draws the symbol of X on a separate sheet of paper and asks each family member, starting with the last one up at the board, to place that symbol as a representation of their greatest frustration.

The facilitator then asks questions and makes appropriate comments about the information obtained by the explanations of the clients about each symbol. Comments from the facilitator are often statements of validation or empathic remarks. Clients placing symbols for their number one concern and deepest frustration usually reveal additional information than that previously identified in the other symbols or even previously mentioned in the forms that clients complete previous to counseling sessions.

Step Eight: Communication Lines

After completing the symbols related to people, environmental factors, stresses, number one concerns, and deepest frustrations, family members are asked to draw communication lines from their own symbol to other symbols that they have drawn within the life space. Mostwin (1980a) describes the lines of communication as a process that moves the interaction between family members and therapists to a deeper level that allows family members to talk about symbols and lines versus painful difficult feelings. Sometimes these lines are not utilized due to time constraints.

The facilitator will instruct each member to draw the line as it relates to how they feel about their communication with each symbol for each person, environmental concern, and stress in the family group. Family members are instructed that they have three options to symbolize communication to the other symbols:

>A solid straight line symbolizes good communication;
>
>A dotted line symbolizes so-so communication;
>
>A line with a slash in it symbolizes poor communication.

Examples of these lines are drawn as examples for the family members. Each family member takes turns drawing the communication lines in their own color.

The facilitator or therapist again makes comments reflective of validating and empathizing with the clients. It is also important sometimes to note differences and similarities when appropriate and as launching pads to the development of the therapeutic process. This is also an opportunity to note incongruences with family positions and lines of communication. An example might be that someone is placed outside the circle but the communication lines are identified as good. This is a chance to reflect on the observation and to ask the client to tell you more about that relationship and the feelings they have connected to that experience. This provides an opportunity for the counselor to learn about the client's thought processes and to offer questions that might help to clarify family connections and relationships.

Step Nine: Reflecting With the Family

After completing all the symbols and the communication lines with the family, it is important to sit back from the drawing and look at the completed picture. Everyone including the therapist has a chance to examine the full picture, which by the time many people have completed it can look pretty chaotic and messy. This is the time to reflect on what family see in the picture. The facilitator might say something similar to this:

> Now that we have completed the drawing, let's review what it was like to complete the drawing and discuss what we see. Now all of this is supposed to have some meaning, but as one of my teachers told me, "All theories are lies in search of truth." Who knows if the theory behind this is correct. I am more interested in what you see and what it was like for you to complete the drawing. What do you notice? What do you see in the family drawing?

Each person is asked to offer comments about completing the drawing and about their experiences related to completing the process. The comments about observing the completed drawing are combined with the already spoken interactive comments previously expressed during the course of each family member placing symbols on the drawing and observing other family members do the same. The ongoing process of asking questions and the interactive discussion of the symbols with each family member while conducting the process actively engages all family members in the process of self-observation (Geddes & Medway, 1977). Each one completing the FLSD becomes an active reporter of the family situation. No one person serves as family spokesperson. The symbolic representations can help family members to observe where they are similar and where they are different.

After people make comments, the therapist has a chance to make their own observations about the family drawing. These reflections should include areas of strengths and positive observations.

It might also include comments about areas of concern or notations about areas to work on in the development of the treatment plan. We also offer some comments related to ways that the FLSD has been interpreted in past observations of other FLSD over the years. At this point in the review of the drawing, clients have chance to agree or disagree with that interpretation and add their own insights.

Mostwin (1980a, p. 17) reflects that the network of relationships is expressed symbolically with the completion of the FLSD, providing a bird's-eye view of the family. Geddes and Medway (1977) reflect that the process of completing this drawing lowers anxiety and reduces blocks to communication. They also suggest that the task obtains family members' attention but also opens the possibility to reveal subconscious information without risking verbal information. Clients and therapists can offer their own interpretations of the visual portrayal of the family.

Step Ten: Developing the Treatment Plan

This final step is the opportunity for creating a joint plan for the future course of treatment. This step is not limited to any one method of working with client groups and can be tailored to each therapist's theoretical model or orientation of working with clients. We suggest that an interactive treatment plan be co-created with the client.

FLSD Symbols

The FLSD uses geometric shapes and straight lines to complete the process. Colors help to identify individuals in the combined process. The following pages illustrate the symbols used in creating the FLSD.

Large Symbol

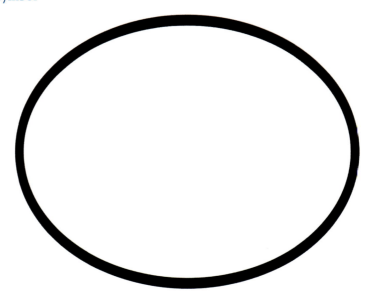

Figure 4.1 Large family symbol

Small Symbol

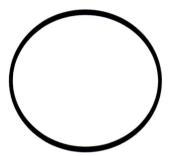

Figure 4.2 Self and significant other symbols

This symbol represents all the people and pets that are part of an individual's history. They include people both currently alive and deceased. They can include biological connections, even if the people never met each other.

Environmental or Institutional Symbol

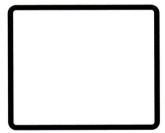

Figure 4.3 Environmental symbols

This symbol represents institutions, organizations, work, social groups, hobbies, and spiritual practices.

Stress Symbol

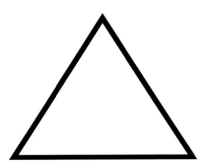

Figure 4.4 Stress symbols

This symbol represents current and past situations that contain emotional significance for the person completing the drawing. This symbol represents areas of stress or concern.

Number One Concern Symbol

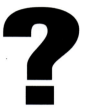

Figure 4.5 Number one concern

This symbol represents the individuals number one concern. This is often a global statement such as peace in the family or a wish that all would be happy

Greatest Frustration Symbol

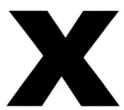

Figure 4.6 Greatest frustration

This symbol describes the greatest frustration at this time. Frustrations often reflect unmet needs, longings, or desires. This symbol is an opportunity to explore these potential issues.

Communication Lines Symbol

Solid lines indicate good communication.

Figure 4.7 Good communication line

Dotted lines indicate so-so communication.

Figure 4.8 So-so communication line

A line with a slash indicates poor communication.

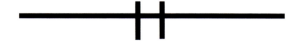

Figure 4.9 Poor communication line

Communication lines help the assessment process in allowing clients to share information about their sense of the relationship between themselves and the persons or places or events in their life space.

Symbolic Representation of the FLSD

The FLSD can be completed in ten steps allowing for obtaining significant information about the family. Through the process of completing the drawing, we learn about:

Family structure;

Family members past and present;

Environmental and institutional factors affecting the family;

Current stressors that are active in the family environment;

Insight into concerns and frustrations;

Communication experiences and feelings around the various components of family relationships.

The FLSD begins the process of client engagement and the development of treatment plans. The FLSD provides hints about the possibility of unconscious information related to self-esteem, family connections, and relationships strengths as well as disconnections in the family system. We gain a little insight into history and family of origin issues affecting all family members. This is most evident in working with couples, as the process helps to identify potential attachment issues. We recognize that not all methods of systemic treatment are interested in obtaining history information. Even so, this process of obtaining information fulfills one of the most important guidelines for assessment, that being joining the client, according to Williams, Edwards, Patterson, and Chamow (2014, p. 9). Completing the FLSD sets the stage for connecting with clients through the sharing of the life story. The FLSD facilitates the process of joining the client in a nonjudgmental, safe manner in a way that is relaxing and interesting for the client to share personal and sometimes difficult information.

Summary

The FLSD involves a ten-step process that includes all of the necessary steps and joining tools to facilitate family assessment and developing the collaborative counseling relationship. The steps include introducing the subject of symbolic meaning in step one. Step two has the facilitator drawing a large symbol for the family. All family members are asked to place themselves in relation to the drawing in step three. Significant others (including pets) are added in step four. Completing the ecological aspect of family assessment involves placing environmental factors in step five and noting stress factors in step six. The drawing can sometimes include optional symbols such as deepest frustration and greatest concern in step seven. The assessment includes drawing communication lines in step eight to represent connection to family members and environmental and stress factors in the family life space. The final steps of the FLSD engage the family by reviewing the drawing in step nine and exploring the experience with the clients and discussing possible insights or observations. In step ten, the family and therapist design and collaboratively complete a treatment plan. The symbolic representations help to begin the therapeutic process between all family members and the connections with the family counselor or therapist.

REFERENCES

Barker, S. B., Barker, R., Dawson, K. S., & Knisely, J. S. (1997). The use of the family life space diagram in establishing interconnectedness: A preliminary study of sexual abuse survivors, their significant others and pets. *Individual Psychology*, 53, 435–450.

Clark, R., Beeton T. (2000). The family Life Space Drawing. Workshop conducted at *International Conference for Imago Relationship Therapy*, Detroit MI.

Geddes, M., & Medway, J. (1977). The symbolic drawing of the family life space. *Family Process*, 16, 219–228.

Ghanbaripanah, A., & Mustaffa, M. S. (2012). The review of family assessment in counseling. *International Journal of Fundamental Psychology & Social Sciences*, 2(2), 32–35

Hartman, A. (1978). Diagrammatic assessment of family relationships. *Social Casework*, 59, 465–476.

Jung, C. J., & Franz, M. V. (1968). *Man and his symbols*. New York, NY: Dell.

Mostwin, D. (1974). The social dimension of family treatment. In D. Mostwin (Ed.), *The social dimension of family treatment* (3rd Annual Seminar). Washington, DC: The Catholic University of America.

Mostwin, D. (1980a). *Social dimension of family treatment*. Washington, DC: National Association of Social Workers Inc.

Mostwin, D. (1980b). Life space approach to the study and treatment of a family. In D. Mostwin (Ed.), *Life space approach to the study and treatment of a family*. Washington, DC: The Catholic University of America.

Mostwin, D. (1982). Predelinquent youth and their families. In D. Mostwin (Ed.), *Ecological therapy: The family life space approach*. Baltimore, MD: Loyola College. Oxford dictionary online retrieved from https://en.oxforddictionaries.com/definition/mandala

Mostwin, D., Clark, R. A., Depenbrock, B. J., McKee, J., & Picado, S. (1977). Short term multidimensional intervention with families in crisis: Use of the therapeutic team. In D. Mostwin (Ed.), *The American family: Continuing impact of ethnicity*. Washington, DC: The Catholic University of America.

Thomlison, B. (2016). *Family assessment handbook: An introduction and practical guide to family assessment* (4th ed.). Boston, MA: Cengage Learning.

Williams, L., Edwards, T. M., Patterson, J., & Chamow, L. (2014). *Essential assessment skills: for couple and family*. New York, NY: Guildford Press.

CHAPTER FIVE
Interpreting the Symbolic Representations of the Family Life Space Drawing

INTERPRETING THE SYMBOLIC REPRESENTATIONS OF THE FLSD

Since developing the FLSD, Mostwin and others began to make observations about the symbolic meaning of the placement, size of symbols, and distances between the symbols in the creation of the family drawing (Mostwin, 1976, 1977; Mostwin, 1980a, 1980b). This chapter will share some of those observations and suggest some starting points for working with clients to understand the message behind the symbolic placements. That being said, we suggest that the best way to discover the meaning of the symbols is to interact and process the significance of the symbols with the clients themselves. We suggest that the placement and size of the symbols will provide some suggestions for providing information on a nonverbal and a visual level. The potential symbolic information gained from clients pertains to placement of symbols, distance between the symbols, size of symbol, and other creative demonstrations developed by the clients.

The first avenue of understanding the FLSD is to explore the presenting obvious message about the symbol. If a person draws a symbol far away from other family members, it is a logical question to pursue information about that representation: "It looks like you see yourself far away from other family members; is that right?" Clients can confirm or deny those conditions and enable the process of learning more about the family situation and interaction.

CONTROL CIRCLE

The control circle developed by Mostwin (1980b, p. 14) provides a framework for discussing observations about the placement of the various symbols used to describe the life space. The control circle uses the concept of a clock and defines symbolic positions as in the 12:00 zone or in the 3:00 zone and so forth. The control zone also provides a reference as to the boundaries related to the family circle. Inquiries and evaluations are made concerning symbols that are in or out of the family life space. The control circle offers a structured concept for understanding the position that people experience themselves in relation to family experiences, with connections to environmental factors and to stresses affecting the family by providing an identifiable frame of reference.

Using the control circle has some limitations due to the lack of standardized paper sizes and family circles, but each larger circle can be the starting point for a frame of reference. The control circle is useful if the regions and clock zones are applied to the size of whatever drawing is being reviewed. It has to be noted that exact notations of where the various zones begin and end will ultimately be left up to the subjective evaluation of the counselor conducting the process. For our purposes, we see the FLSD as having three zones that provide references for understanding all the persons in the life space. For our purpose, we used a compass to create the various circles all with increasing size: 1.5 for inner, 2.5 for middle, and 3.5 for outer as an example of the demonstrated examples.

The control circle has been divided into three zones, inner, middle, and outer zones.

Mostwin (1980b, p. 13) made some observations that certain positions in the FLSD have symbolic meaning concerning the experiences of all of the individuals in the family. Clark and Beeton also provide some observations from their use of the process in the last 40-plus years. The zones once again provide a starting point for understanding the family.

INNER ZONE

Usually placement in the inner zone signifies an emotional and expressive position. Clark and Beeton have identified the central zone as holding the heart of the family. This inner zone is often occupied by parents in a family and by spouses in a drawing completed by couples when all is functioning in a connected fashion. Individuals with good ego strength will often place themselves in the center of the circle. People will often place pets in the

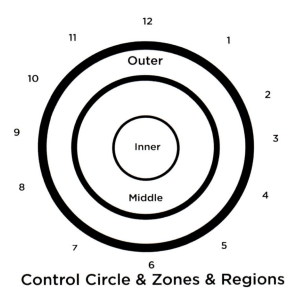

Figure 5.1 Control circle, zones, and regions

center, possibly reflecting deep emotional connection. Mostwin noted that the middle position of the inner zone often symbolizes a sense of responsibility and emotional value (Mostwin, 1976, 1980a).

Middle Zone

The middle zone of the circle shows connection to the inner circle, but without the deeper emotional connection of the inner circle. Placement in the middle zone can often indicate a more neutral experience without strong positive or negative emotions. Placements in this zone do not necessarily raise concerns but need to be investigated in the interactive process of meeting the client.

Outer Zone

Mostwin (1980a, p. 62) indicates that the upper outer circle between the hours of 10:00 and 2:00 is considered a position of dominance and authority in families. Clark and Beeton have noted that this position also indicates a position of significance and can be either negative or positive. To offer a mirror opposite to the position of authority and dominance, the lower part of the control circle between the hours of 8:00 and 4:00 are considered positions of low self-esteem or for persons with a sense of rejection. Sometimes this position is occupied by people who want to disconnect or reject emotional involvement with the family. It also is often held by people with a sense of no power or low value in the family system. (Barker, Barker, Dawson, Knisely, 1997) noticed that survivors of childhood sexual abuse recalled their childhood by placing themselves low in the outer circle or on the edge of it.

People often draw people, environmental factors, and stress factors that are less important to them in the lower quadrants. Placing these symbols in the lower quadrants may be a situation when clients want to indicate an unfavorable or distasteful sense of the person, environmental, or stress factor. Or it could be that placement in this area may just be an indication that the symbol has less meaning to the person drawing the symbol.

Other Placements

Our observations reveal that sometimes people place family members and other life space factors outside the circle. When people place themselves in this position, it usually indicates that the person does not feel like they are a part of the family. When people place other family members outside the circle, usually they are indicating a sense of cutoff with that part of the person's life. People often place past love relationships outside the family circle. Other serious indicators of family cutoffs and disconnections are people who place themselves partially in the circle and partially out of the circle. This placement indicates ambivalence as to staying in the family or reveals a sense of uncertainty and is often seen by marital couples uncertain of their commitment to their marital situation. Young adults making a transition to their own adulthood sometimes present this type of picture. We have also observed placements of symbols on the edge of the family circle. We draw conclusions supported by some research (Barker & Barker, 1990); Barker, Barker, Dawson, & Knisely,

1997) that distance from the family or self indicates a lack of relationship and closeness. Symbols placed outside the family circle appear to be less connected to the person placing the symbol in that area.

Research still needs to provide more details about the meaning of placement in the various zones of the life space.

Placement of Symbols

Client placement in the FLSD can reveal information about sense of self-esteem and their sense of their role and function as a family member in the family group. Symbol placement can reveal information about the significance and relationships of whatever symbol is being drawn. The interactive process of completing the FLSD provides a vehicle for exploring hypothetical assumptions concerning symbolic placements.

Clark (2002) expresses an observation that looking at the whole picture reveals information concerning family trends and connections. Clark looks for the way that family individuals represent their symbols and observes how family members locate their symbols either in separate sections of the drawing or all over the circle. The FLSD can reveal if a member of the family group lives in an isolated world or in an integrated life space environment. An example of this would be observing clusters of colors. Since each person has their own marker and color, the drawing shows whether the person occupies one section or not. Clustered drawings can reveal isolation. The use of the colored markers also helps to identify if family members show the same value for similar environmental factors. An example of this issue would be observing the placement of an environmental factor, such as church. Some family members can place the factor high and other family members can place the factor low. Placement can reveal that people see things in a similar fashion or from different perspectives. Placement of environmental factors can indicate the emotional impact of the factor. If the factor has high placement or surrounds the circle, it provides information as to the impact of that factor on the individual or family placing the symbol.

Other observations concerning placement pertain to where people place others in relationship to themselves. Most people generally do not draw circles over other people. People drawing significant others with circle overlapping or intersecting may indicate too much emotional closeness. Such emotional closeness can reveal a potential for mental illness (Clark & Beeton, 2000). If the FLSD has a lot of overlapping symbols, it is important to investigate the underlying aspects of those intersections if possible.

Observing the areas of placements in the FLSD can reveal information about family organization and hierarchy. Placements of circles above and below the person reveals information about emotional connections and sense of self in relationship to others. Usually we see symbols placed above the self, showing respect or importance, whereas symbols below the self might show less respect or low importance, depending on placement. If a person places a parent or grandparent below them, it might be an indication of poor connections or the presence of current custodial relationship for that grandparent. If people place minor children in position of power or in positions above them, it may indicate that children are operating in dominant positions. It would be important to explore family culture and norms to discover if placements are congruent with family expectations. Therapists need to inquire about role expectations and discover if the family follows a traditional family structure and if the family is satisfied or discouraged with current family structure.

Distances and Closeness

Mostwin (1980a) reports that the most telling part of the FLSD is the message revealed by the placement of the family members in relation to each other. The zones can provide some insight into the functioning of individuals in the family system, but the placement of the people in relation to each other reveals information about family connectedness. When investigating the construct validity of the FLSD, Barker and Barker (1990) discovered that when individuals described relationships with words such as being close and connected, they were likely to draw the symbols closer to them. In subsequent research, Barker et al. (1997) were able to discover that childhood sexual abuse survivors placed abusers on the opposite side of their own placements in a faraway, distant position.

Size of Symbol

The size of the symbol used in the FLSD is a possible indicator for how the person drawing the symbol experiences the item they are reflecting on. When instructing on how to indicate a symbol reflective of themselves and significant people, environmental elements, or stress factors in their current life, clients are given a sample drawing by the facilitator. Usually the example is a smaller circle on a separate page. When clients are creating the symbol, they will often take the opportunity to draw a size that comes from their own perspectives and experiences and draw something either very large or very small. We recognize the projective process of this component, as clients show personal initiative to create their own symbols and placements.

The size and placement of the symbol for people may be an indication of self-esteem or individual regard for the item being represented. Individuals who draw large symbols in relation to others may indicate a sense of grandiosity or overimportance. The reverse is true for individuals who draw smaller circles in relation to others. Small circles can possibly indicate a level of low self-esteem or low levels of responsibility in the family system. One person who presented as clinically depressed drew themselves the size of a marker dot. The depressed person drew other family members as significantly larger than their own symbol. The majority of people draw circles similar to the example given to them by the facilitator of the process or will make the symbols similar to their own symbol in size. Another observation concerning the symbols for people relates to whether or not the person drawing the symbol completes the circle. Incomplete circles can be an indication of unfinished business concerning the person symbolically represented.

The notation of the size of the symbol applies to all of the symbols used in the FLSD. Large squares indicate that the factor takes a lot of energy and time. Some people draw work as a square that covers the whole circle. This is a possible indication that the person's work overrides the family. The same situation exists with the size of symbols related to stress. People experiencing a greater sense of stress with multiple stresses will reveal one large stress symbol, even to the point of drawing a large triangle over the family circle. The same situation holds true for smaller symbols. Small symbols may represent that the factor is not that significant in the family life space. An example might be that low levels of stress get represented as small symbols.

Interpreting Number One Concern and Greatest Frustration Symbols

The use of the "X" and "?" symbols provide the therapist with an opportunity to learn more about the unconscious issues of the client or client group. Participants of the FLSD are able to represent the concern or frustration and discuss it with the therapist. Placement and size of the symbol help the therapist to know more about the person's experience of the issue. Large symbols indicate strong emotions and experiences. The placement of the symbol follows similar patterns of the other symbols. Symbols placed close to the person drawing the FLSD reveal a more intense connection with the issue. The use of this symbol also helps to identify presenting issues or concerns for therapy. Family members are able to show separate or combined concerns. The identification of frustrations and concerns helps clients and therapist to develop conjoint treatment plans. Ronald A. Clark (2002) developed the use of this symbol in order to expand the information about stresses within the individuals in the couple or family.

It is always useful to ask people in the process of drawing the FLSD to give feedback concerning the information they reveal. It is most useful to ask the clients involved in the process to provide their own interpretation of the placements. The clients' experience can provide important information in understanding the true meaning of the symbolic placements. The interactive dynamic of the process allows for the therapist to keep on investigating any symbolic representation that does not instinctively feel congruent with what the therapist is seeing or hearing.

All of these observations concerning the significance of symbolic placement require some systematic validation through a structured research process. We are hopeful that the future will be able to test out our observations as having some validity. In the meantime, we use our observations and interactions with specific clients, couples, and families to provide feedback and discussion about possible meanings applied by the client to the symbolic placement and its relation to self and family.

The basic premise operating in using the FLSD is to obtain projective and preconscious information while obtaining conscious information (Mostwin, 1980a). The process of conducting the FLSD provides basic information such as family constellations, occupation, spiritual orientation, social affiliations, activities, and community involvement. The FLSD has the opportunity to reveal more information concerning the relationship of the person to the people and environmentally connections affecting the individual, such as noticing symbols placed at a distance or in a high or low location. Interpretation of the FLSD relies on a theoretical foundation that clients will symbolically project onto the drawing information pertaining to self-esteem and a sense of emotional connections to persons and environmental factors in the client's life.

Obtaining Client Information With the FLSD

The FLSD process is a good starting point for most types of family counseling. The process can identify most information that is normally gathered in initial intake sessions. In addition, the process can provide information about deeper issues related to the development of treatment plans. The following outline presents an indication of the potential for information that the FLSD process can obtain. FLSD provides the following information for initial appointments:

I. Identifying information

   A. Family composition

      1. All persons both sharing and absent from the family household

      2. Identifying information about extended family including parents, grandparents, and significant others

B. Family social characteristics
   1. Age, education, occupation: immediate and extended family
   2. Spiritual background and present experience
   3. Geographic family information, past and present
   4. Local family support
   5. Primary institutional factors
   6. Current stresses

II. Family dynamics and structure
   A. Position and placement of individuals relative to the family life space in relation to others by identifying zone of placement
   B. Indicate size of symbols drawn by each participant
   C. Indicate patterns of communication and quality of communication between family members and significant others within and outside the home
   D. Connections to institutional factors and stresses indicated by size placement and communication lines

III. Potential counseling issues and treatment goals
   A. Identify patterns from FLSD to determine efforts toward effective differentiation and healthy connection
   B. Assist with appropriate management of relationships, institutional factors, and stresses
   C. Improve or reinforce effective communications and connections

Ideal Family Representations

Sometimes in the process of discussing family drawings with clients, we show them a representation of what we look for in healthy family functioning. It is mentioned that ideal drawings rarely are demonstrated. These "ideal" representations also portray the traditional Western family structure. We recognize that this understanding does not work for all models of knowing families, and we encourage both the facilitator and family members to identify what healthy functioning means to them in their own constructs of understanding.

The potential ideal position in the FLSD will show people drawing themselves in the center of the circle. The following understanding of healthy functioning follows a traditional Western path of understanding more common in the original models of family therapy's understanding of systems theory. The center of the circle indicates emotional connections and sense of responsibility (Mostwin, 1980a). Parents often place themselves in the center of the circle when both parents operate in a cohesive parenting relationship. If one partner in a marriage places themselves outside the center, it could be a sign that they do not operate in a parental role, either by abdication or a sense of rejection. An example of healthy family functioning will show parents in the center, with minor children slightly lower but still in the inner zone of the circle. Parents of the parents will hold a slightly higher position, and the great grandparents will hold a slightly higher position. This type of drawing might indicate that family connections were basically healthy and that the family experienced little or no emotional cutoffs from previous generations.

IDEAL PLACEMENTS

The following is a graphic example of a two-person drawing. The only symbols examined are placement of people. The example shows an example of symbols in a balanced or healthy drawing. Other symbols for environment and stress are not included in this example.

REPRESENTING IDEAL FAMILY PLACEMENTS: CASE EXAMPLE 5.A

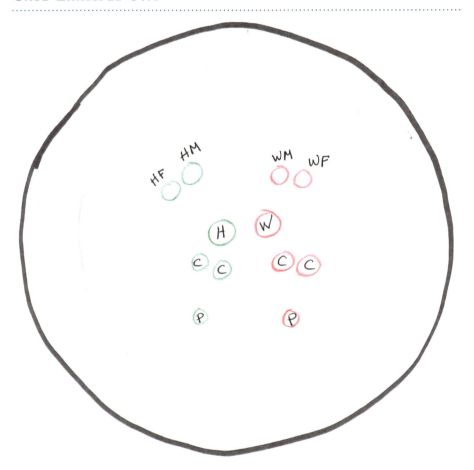

Figure 5.2 Example of ideal placements in FLSD

This drawing shows parents in the center. The wife is the red center circle, and the husband is the green center circle. The mother places two children slightly below in red circles. The husband represents the two children in green circles slightly below his circle. Both parents

INTERPRETING SYMBOLIC REPRESENTATIONS | 59

place their own parents above them in their own colors. All of the symbols are close to the emotional center. The symbols are not too small or too big. The symbols show connection and a continuing sense of family that shows little or no emotional cutoffs. Notice that family members are located close to the center. Notice the family pet in the lower inner circle.

The ideal representation allows the therapist to operate with a starting point. The ideal symbolic representation provides an opportunity to gauge family or couple closeness and to learn about the presence or lack of presence of family connections. Considering the ideal representation is an opportunity to explore how the family in the room compares with ideal connections. We note what appears to be strengths in family relationships, such as reflecting to clients in the drawing process, "you are located in the center it looks like you really care about your family." We also note areas of disconnection or difficult experiences in family, such as: "It appears you are located outside the family circle; that looks lonely." Symbolic drawings actually reveal a combination of factors and rarely present in a neat and orderly fashion even when presenting a close to ideal situation. Most symbolic drawings can look chaotic and messy when all the symbols are in place, no matter if they show positive or negative family situations.

CASE EXAMPLE 5.B WITH SYMBOLIC INTERPRETATION

The following example is from a couple seeking relationship counseling. The wife is 38 years old and the husband is 40 years old. They have been married for 12 years and have two children. The couple is American, Caucasian, and both have European ancestry. They are self-considered middle class. The wife's parents divorced when she was a teenager. She has one older sister and one younger brother. She had a relationship with both sets of grandparents. Her maternal grandparents died before she married her husband. The wife currently holds a full-time job. She has a hobby of exercising at a fitness club. She sometimes attends a Protestant church in the denomination that she knew from her childhood. She expresses her frustrations as concerns about herself and making decisions about her life. She expresses a frustration concerning her current relationship with her husband. She also identified a stress concerning her relationship with her father. She expresses stress concerning her husband's family. Her number one concern is to "make sure that everything in life works out all right." Her greatest frustration is that her relationship and life are not working out.

The husband in the drawing comes from a family where both parents remained married. His mother is currently deceased and died in the last few years from cancer. His father lives nearby. The husband has two younger brothers. He knew his grandparents, but they are deceased. He has a full-time job. He identifies a hobby of sometimes playing golf. He sometimes attends the Protestant church with his wife, but he has a different denominational background. The husband identifies his stresses related to his work, concerns about relationship, and finances. He states that his number one concern is that he takes care of his family. His greatest frustration is that his wife is unhappy.

The following example will follow a couples completing the FLSD and review it in stages to match how the drawing and symbols evolve in the process of completing all the symbols and what they show at the time they are created. The example starts from step three, showing placements for self, and then moves to step four, showing placement of self and significant family members. The example will continue with step five, adding environmental factors, and continue with another example of step six that adds the symbols for stresses, and then show a drawing including step seven, which shows symbols for number one concern and greatest frustration.

STEP THREE: PLACEMENT OF SELF

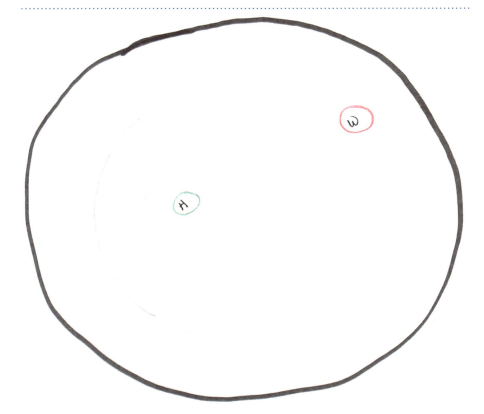

Figure 5.3 Step three: placement of self, Example 5.B

Table 5.1 Placement zone, region, size, and distance, Example 5.A

Wife: red	Husband: green
Zone and region: middle and outer between 2:00 and 3:00	**Zone and region**: inner zone 3:00
Size: Average size	**Size**: Average size
Distance: 6 cm from center, 6.8 from spouse	**Distance**: 1.6 cm from center

The wife is located partially in the middle and outer zone of the family circle. Her position might be indicating a movement away from the emotional center of the relationship. Sometimes this position is an indication that the partner is on the way to exiting the relationship. She is placed in the higher positions, close to 2:00 – a possible indication of good self-esteem.

The husband in this drawing places himself close to the emotional center in the inner zone in the 3:00 region. This placement of the male spouse is a possible indication that he is more invested in working on this relationship.

Step Four: Placement of Significant Others

Key to Symbols

Wife, red	Husband, blue
W: wife	H: husband
M: mother	M: mother
F: father	F: father
C: children	C: children
P: pet	P: pet
B: brother	B1: brother 1
S: sister	B2: brother 2
MGM: maternal grandmother	MGM: maternal grandmother
MGF: maternal grandfather	MGF: Maternal grandfather
PGF: paternal grandfather	PGM paternal grandmother
PGM: paternal grandmother	PGF paternal grandfather

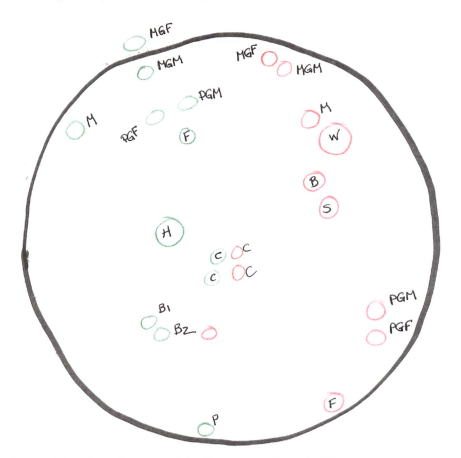

Figure 5.4 Step four: placement of significant others, Example 5.B

Table 5.2 Significant others: zone and region, Example 5.B

Wife: red	Husband: green
Outside: no symbols	**Outside:** MGF-11:00 region
Outer: F, 5:00 region	**Outer:** MGM, 11:00 region
MGF, 12:00 region	M, between 9:00 an 10:00
PGF, 4:00	P, 6:00
PGM, partial	
Middle: M, 2:00	**Middle:** PGF, 11:00
B, partial 2:00	PGM, between 11:00 and 12:00
S, partial 3:00	F, 11:00
PGM, partial 4:00	B1 and B2, 7:00
Inner: C and C, center 3:00	**Inner:** C and C, center 3:00
B, partial 2:00	
S, partial 3:00	
P, 6:00	

Table 5.3 Significant others: size and distance, Example 5.B

Wife: red	Husband: green
Size: sizes are similar to each other	**Size:** size of symbols similar to each other
Distance:	**Distance:**
M 1 cm; S 1 cm; B 1 cm	M 5.2 cm; F 2.7 cm
C 4.6 cm; C 5.2 cm	C 1.5 cm; C 2 cm
PGM 4.7 cm; PGF 6 cm	B1 3.5 cm; B2 4 cm
MGM 4.4 cm; MGF 5.5 cm	PGM 4.3 cm; PGF 3.8 cm
F 8 cm	MGM 5.6 cm; MGF 7 cm
P 8.5 cm	P 6.8 cm

Reflections on Wife's Placements

The mother of the wife is located above her between the middle and outer zone. Father is located in lower section edge of the circle near the 5:00 position. The parents' divorce is reflected in the distance between the parents. Children are placed in the inner zone. Siblings are located close to her in the middle and inner zone, with sister located closer than the brother. The placement of these symbols might indicate a cutoff with father and a sense of respect for mother. Children are located in the emotional center of the family. Maternal grandparents are in a place of respect and authority. Paternal grandparents are in outer ring of the circle and in the lower middle zone section of the drawing just above her father. This might be a clue as to disconnections with that side of the family. She places her symbols for significant people on the right side of the drawing.

The sizes of symbols are relatively the same and do not reflect indications of being overwhelmed by any of the people.

The wife's most distant symbols are to her father and her family pet. The closest symbols are her mother and sister and brother. The children have some distance but their location in the emotional center shows that they have a significant position in the family. The wife's placements begin to suggest her family background and disconnections with her father. She shows some potential support with siblings and mother.

Reflections on Husband's Placements

The husband has placed his children near him in the inner circle just below him. His father is placed above him in the middle zone. His mother is located on the outer edge of the circle, close to the 10:00 position. Her position reflects some disconnect. We do note that she has recently died, and this position may be related to a long-term illness and the difficulties of caregiving and relating to a seriously ill person. His paternal grandparents are located above his father in the middle zone of the circle at the 11:00 position. The maternal grandmother is in the outer zone, with the maternal grandfather on the outside of the family life space symbol. The location of maternal grandparents might indicate some cutoffs or difficult experiences with this part of the family. The family pet is located in the outer circle in a lower position, possibly indicating that he is not as connected to the pet or has had some difficult experiences with the animal. He locates his symbols for significant people on the left side of the drawing.

The size of the symbols related to people are not remarkably large or small. No one symbol seems larger than another.

He locates himself 5.2 cm from his mother's symbol and 2.7 cm from his father's symbol. His closest symbols are with his children: one child is 1.5 cm and the other is 2 cm. His most distant symbol, 7 cm, is connected to his maternal grandfather on the outside of the family circle. The family pet is almost as distant, at 6.8 cm. As previously noted, the distance between spouses is 6.8 cm. Please note that spouses do not draw each other at the time of the FLSD. His brothers are located in the lower middle zone and may or may not be a source of support, as demonstrated by a 3.5 and 4 cm distance in the lower location. The husband's placements in this drawing indicate some disconnects with his mother and maternal grandmother.

The evaluation of this couple will continue by taking the original drawing that placed self and significant people and add environmental factors to the symbolic placement of people.

Step five involves adding environmental factors. In this case, each has placed work, children's school, hobbies, and spiritual practice.

STEP FIVE: ENVIRONMENTAL SYMBOLS

Key to Symbols

Wife's symbols in red　　**Husband's symbols in green**

W: work
CS: children's sports
E: exercise
C: church
HW: husband's work
HH: Husband's hobbies

W: work
H: hobbies
C: church

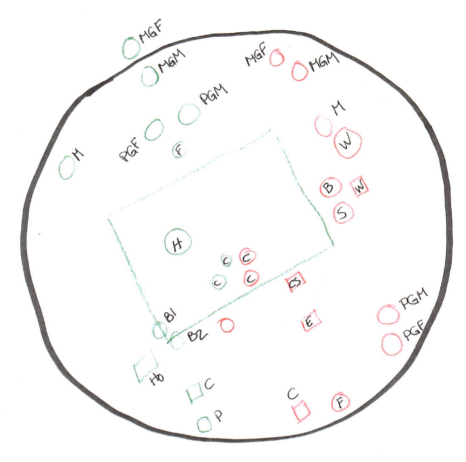

Figure 5.5 Step five: environmental symbols, Example 5.B

Table 5.4 Environmental symbols: zones, region, size, and distance, Example 5.B

Wife: red	Husband: green
Outside: no symbols	**Outside:** no symbols
Outer: C 5:00	**Outer:** C 6:00, H partial 7:00
Middle: E 5:00; W 3:00	
Inner: CS 7:00; HH 6:00; HW 9:00	**Inner:** W 12:00–7:00; 9:00–3:00
Size: size similar to all other symbols but smaller than self-symbol	**Size:** extra-large symbol for W; other symbols smaller than symbols for self
Distance: CS 4.5 cm; E 4 cm; W 1 cm HH 5.8 cm; HW 7.7 cm	**Distance:** W no distance, engulfs his symbol C 7.5 cm; H 5.6 cm

Reflections on Wife's Environmental Symbols

Wife places her work straddling the middle zone just below her symbol. She places the symbol related to her church in the lowest part of the circle, indicating a position of less importance or the possibility of negative feelings toward this symbol. She places exercise as a hobby in the middle zone but lower in the family circle. The wife places symbols related to children's school near the children but below them in the inner circle—possibly symbolizing emotional value to the family. She places husband's work above the husband in the emotional center of the family. His hobbies are located below the husband but all in the emotional center.

The size of the environmental symbols does not show a remarkable indication and appears to be in proportion to other factors in the life space.

The closest environmental symbol in this drawing is the wife's work. That symbol is 1 cm. The most distant symbol is the church, which is 7.6 cm. This distance might indicate that her experience with the church is not a source of support for her. The symbols that are also distant from her are symbols connected to husband and his activities. These activities all fall in the 5.8 cm to 7.7 cm range. Children's school is also 7 cm (note is it located in inner zone). The children's sports are also a closer distance, located at 4.5 cm. What this might be revealing is that she has some distance from the inner workings of family life and could possibly be attempting to disconnect from these actions. These are important considerations to investigate.

The symbolic indications on the environmental level indicate that her symbols are distant from her and that she is most close to her sense of employment. She places most of her personal symbols in the lower section of the life space. Many of these indicators need to be investigated as to her own level of involvement with children's activities.

Reflections on Husband's Environmental Symbols

The husband places his symbol for work in the emotional center of the family. This symbol surrounds him and other symbols near the inner circle center. The symbol intersects symbols for his brothers, and we discover that his brothers have a similar business. He places his hobbies in the lower outer circle along with his symbol for spiritual practice. He had three symbols for his own interests. He does not place symbols for his children's activities or for his wife's activities.

The most striking symbol in this drawing is connected to the symbol for his work. We would guess that he has an absorbing job and that it requires a lot of time and energy. We discover that he does have his own business and that he has much responsibility for the day-to-day activities and the business success. Other symbols do not demonstrate as significant impact in the family life space.

There is no distance between himself and work, and in fact work engulfs him. He has his spiritual practice as the most distant symbol, 7.5 cm, and his hobby also in a distant place, at 5.6 cm. As he remarks in the process," I do not have much time for hobbies."

The symbol for work is the most remarkable aspect of this drawing, and it would be important to find out more about his occupation and the place it takes in his life experiences. This symbol provides a visual reference into exploring this symbol's connection to marital stress and disconnection. It would also be important to note the symbols that were missing in this drawing. The facilitator needs to inquire about symbols that are forgotten or inadvertently not drawn. We encourage the addition of missing symbols.

STEP SIX: STRESS SYMBOLS

Key to Symbols

Wife	**Husband**
S: self	R: relationship
C: children	W: work
R: relationship	F: finances
HF: his family	
F: issues with father	

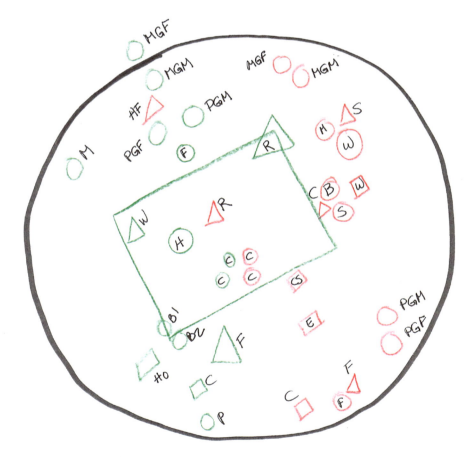

Figure 5.6 Step six: stress symbols, Example 5.B

Table 5.5 Step six, stress symbols: zone, region, size, and distance, Example 5.B

Wife: red	Husband: green
Outside: no symbols	**Outside:** no symbols
Outer: F 5:00; S partial 2:00 HF, 11:00	**Outer:** no symbols
Middle: S partial 2:00	**Middle:** F 6:00 partial; W 9:00
Inner: C 3:00; R 3:00	**Inner:** R 12:00 partial; W 9:00
Size: symbols are smaller than symbol for self	**Size:** symbols for F and R are largest
Distance: C 1.9 cm; S 0.2 cm; R 5.6 cm HF 9.4 cm; F 5.3 cm	**Distance:** F 4.5 cm; W 1.2 cm R 2.5 cm

Reflections on Wife's Stress Symbols

The wife has a symbol for stress above herself. This symbol is near her partially in the outer and middle zone. She places a symbol inside the inner circle near the symbol that the husband placed for himself. She also places a stress symbol touching the husband's work symbol, representing the children. She also has a stress symbol in the lower outer zone depicting stress issues with her father. She places a stress symbol near his maternal grandmother in the outer zone. The size of these symbols in this category are relatively small.

Her closest symbol is to her stress about herself, about 0.2 cm. This is located near her in the outer and middle zone. The stress symbol for her father is about 5.3 cm away from her own symbol located near her symbol for her father in the outer zone. Stress with her marital relationship is 5.6 cm and is located in the inner circle. The stress symbol with his family is 9.4 cm and is located in the outer zone. The stress symbol related to children is 1.9 cm and is located in the inner circle.

The closest stress symbols are connected to herself and the children. We would guess that the symbols show us a struggle to manage her internal conflicts. Inner zone stresses connect to children and the relationship. There are some hints of family of origin and in-law issues. Clients will usually provide information to determine if therapy needs to consider these areas.

Reflections on Husband's Stress Symbols

Stress symbols placed in inner zone are connected to work. He has two symbols in the middle zone connected to his relationship and concern for finances. The relationship stress symbol is placed above him toward the right outer zone.

The size of his stress symbol for relationship is his largest symbol, with finances being close in size. Interestingly his stress symbol for work is not as large. This might indicate that he can manage this stress.

The closest stress symbol is the one for work, 1.2 cm. His stress symbol for his relationship is 2.5 cm, and his stress symbol for finances is the most distant, being located 4.5 cm away from his symbol for self.

There were only three stress symbols. The largest symbol concerns his relationship and might signify this issue as an important concern to him. The placement of this symbol in the inner zone also reflects the significance of this concern to the husband.

Table 5.6 Step seven, optional symbols: number one concern (?) and greatest frustration (X), Example 5.B

Wife: red	Husband: green
?: middle zone, 2:00, similar size close to her own symbol, 0.6 cm	?: inner zone, 3:00, close to his own symbol, 0.6 cm
X: inner zone center near symbol for children similar in size, 4.2 cm from her symbol	X: middle zone, 2:00 region, near his wife's symbols for family, 6 cm from his symbol

STEP SEVEN: NUMBER ONE CONCERN AND GREATEST FRUSTRATION SYMBOLS

Wife's Placement for Symbol of Number One Concern and Greatest Frustration

The wife's symbol for number one concern represented by a question mark was placed near her own symbol. The wife reported that her number one concern is to "make sure that everything in life works out all right." It is located in the middle zone next to her symbol on the lower left.

The symbol for her greatest frustration represented by a large X mark is located in the center of the inner circle of the drawing. She reports that her greatest frustration is that "her relationship and her life is not working out." She places this symbol near her symbol for her children.

These symbols connect to what we have been seeing in the previous stages of the drawing. Distance between the wife is evident in the placing of her symbols and the family center.

Husband's Placement for Symbol of Number One Concern and Greatest Frustration

The husband placed his symbol for his number one concern near his own symbol located in the inner zone. The symbol as reported by the husband represents his number one concern, to take care of his family.

The symbol for greatest frustration is located in the middle zone to the left of his wife's symbol that she placed for herself. He reports that his greatest frustration is that his wife is unhappy.

The choice for the placement of these symbols are confirming of the other symbols and placements in this FLSD. The husband has a large focus on work and his number one concern relates to taking care of his family (we might infer that means financially). His symbol for his greatest frustration concerning his wife's unhappiness fits with its placement near her symbol.

POSSIBLE USES OF THIS INFORMATION WITH CASE EXAMPLE 5.B

The most significant way to use this information with a couple is to allow the couple to reflect on the picture itself. It is useful to ask couples to reflect on what they see and what

INTERPRETING SYMBOLIC REPRESENTATIONS | 69

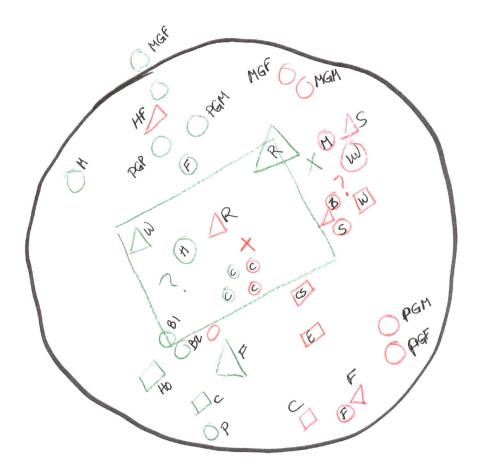

Figure 5.7 Step seven: greatest concern and frustration, Example 5.B

they learned and what they experienced about themselves from completing the FLSD. The therapist could ask questions about family relationships and expectations about relationship. The therapist could report that "It looks like you have some distance from your mother or father; tell me more about that." Clients can confirm or deny and fill in the gaps with more information. The FLSD informs the therapist that this couple has great emotional distance between each other. The hopeful expression in the picture is that both members place some significant symbols in the center.

The FLSD drawing gives the therapist a heads up about possible sources of trouble or exits in the relationship such as the husband's job. It also informs about possible sources of help if close family members are present or not present. The FLSD reveals intergenerational relationship patterns, such as in this case divorce, emotional cutoffs, and disconnects.

The couple has an opportunity to reflect on ways that they would like to change family patterns. The therapist can point to the drawing and ask the wife to work on coming back to the emotional center. The therapist might say: "Would you be willing to make it a goal of therapy to work on improving the connection between husband and wife?" The symbolic representations in the FLSD also provide an opportunity to design goals of therapy. Therapists and clients can reflect on the stress symbols and the symbols of their number one concern and greatest frustrations in deciding goals.

The symbolic drawing of the family life space allows the client to share information on a conscious and preconscious level. The example couple provides information about the make-up of their family including information concerning the emotional distance between themselves and other family members. The FLSD provides information concerning environmental factors including hobbies and work. The drawing also starts the conversation around stress factors and previously unspoken words about concerns and frustrations.

Summary

The symbols used in the FLSD can help therapist and clients to understand the family situation by providing not only verbal information but also visual information about the family situation. Throughout the years of utilizing the FLSD in various counseling practices, ideas about the meaning of the symbols has developed. These possible considerations about size, placement, and distances between symbols is a launching pad for counseling inquiry. Counselors working with the family can ask questions about the symbols and offer some possible ideas from past interpretations used by the developers and past practitioners of the FLSD.

References

Barker, S. B., & Barker, R. T. (1990). Investigation of the construct validity of the family life space diagram. *Journal of Mental Health Counseling*, 12, 506–514.

Barker, S. B., Barker, R. T., Dawson, K. S., & Knisley, J. S. (1997). The use of the family life space diagram in establishing interconnectedness: A preliminary study of sexual abuse survivors, their significant others, and pets. *Individual Psychology*, 53, 433–450.

Clark, R. (2002). *Interpretation of the life space drawing*. Handout at Workshop: Family Life Space Drawing.

Clark, R., & Beeton, T. (2000). *The family life space drawing*. Workshop Conducted at International Conference for Imago Relationship Therapy, Detroit, MI.

Mostwin, D. (1976). The social dimension of family treatment. In D. Mostwin (Ed.), *The social dimension of family treatment* (3rd Annual Seminar). Washington, DC: The Catholic University of America.

Mostwin, D. (1977). Social work intervention with families in crisis of change. In D. Mostwin (Ed.), *The social dimension of treatment: The American family: Continuing impact of ethnicity*. Washington, DC: The Catholic University of America.

Mostwin, D. (1980a). *Social dimension of family treatment*. Washington, DC: National Association of Social Workers.

Mostwin, D. (1980b). Life space approach to the study and treatment of a family. In D. Mostwin (Ed.), *Life space approach to the study and treatment of a family*. Washington, DC: The Catholic University of America.

PART TWO

Using the Family Life Space Drawing (FLSD) With Different Types of Clients

INTRODUCTION

We have facilitated the completion of thousands of Family Life Space drawings and have seen the value of engaging all types of clients with this process and using it with any theoretical orientation of working with clients in therapy. The FLSD can be a useful process when developing counseling relationships with individuals, couples, and families. We have even utilized the concept when working with groups and organizations.

The following chapters will provide case examples of using the FLSD with different types of clients. The examples in Chapter 6 concern FLSDs drawn by people participating in an individual counseling session. Chapter 7 illustrates examples of couples seeking marital or relationship counseling, and Chapter 8 demonstrates FLSDs completed with multiple family members. Chapter 9 will demonstrate with case examples how the FLSD has been used with specific client groups in various counseling settings. The final chapter in the book will include a discussion of past research and share some examples of pilot study research comparisons of the FLSD with standard relationship measures.

The exploration of the examples of FLSDs with individuals, couples, and families will include a brief review of the presenting problem and identifying information about the case example. The examples with include illustrations of the drawing and provide an analysis of the drawing as it evolves in the various steps of completing the drawing. To complete the analysis the presentation will discuss how to use the drawing with example and a discussion of the emerging outcomes of treatment.

None of the examples are from specific clients and the examples portray composites of the drawings we have witnessed over the years of facilitating these drawings with different types of clients. The examples portray some of potential possibilities of what people might present when completing a FLSD. These composite examples will provide insight on what facilitator might see while completing the FLSD. Each drawing is a unique representation of the client's life space and is always a very interesting finished product.

The examples of drawings in these chapters are hand-drawn to give as close an example as we can to the experience of the drawing with a client. Oftentimes the image of the original symbol for the family circle is not as even or an exact circle when we draw the image on the easel board. These example drawings also include the designations drawn with faint lines in the background of the symbol for the control circle regions. In a typical FLSD these lines will not be available to the view of the client. We provide these lines in an effort to help with the examination and understanding of the various drawings while learning how to view them. We do not suggest that the FLSD include the region and zones on the papers set aside to complete a FLSD. Clients need to view a blank paper that gradually includes the original large circle signifying the family boundary. The view of the drawing will gradually include symbols for self, significant others, and environmental factors as well as symbols for stress. Communication lines maybe included along with symbols for greatest concern and deepest frustration.

We present the analysis of the information in terms of how the clients place their symbols by identifying the region and zone of the placement and noting the size of the symbol. The analysis also includes a listing of the distances between the symbols for self and significant others as identified and placed in the drawing. While measuring distance between the symbols has some potential for understanding connections and relationships between the symbols it is more valuable to review the whole picture of the drawing to analyze how the people in the family view their connection to each other. The holistic view of the family members in relation to each other will be the best illumination as to actual family functioning. We recognize that measuring distance between the symbols provides some limited information about client connections with other family members, environmental factors, and stress issues within the life space. Even so, it is important to include other information when viewing the whole picture. We look for the holistic view of the drawing or the bird's-eye view of the drawing. People may place symbols at a distance from their symbol but place the other symbols in a significant place, such as the center or in the positions of respect and authority. All of those conditions must be taken into account when evaluating and making determinations about the meaning of the drawing.

Part Two will allow the reader to obtain a view of how we the authors have analyzed and utilized the FLSD. We encourage our colleagues to explore the potential use of the FLSD with their own clients and in their own settings.

CHAPTER SIX
The Individual Family Life Space Drawing

The Individual FLSD

Completing an individual life space drawing with a client can serve many useful purposes. Individual client drawings will provide the therapist with client-specific knowledge about the people in the family system and inform on the ecological aspects of the whole family life space. Completing a FLSD is a vehicle for obtaining some insight as to the client's own experience of being in their specific life. The drawing has the potential to be a holistic process in that it not only reveals information about family and social connections but also informs on potential insights as to the experience of that person to environmental factors and stresses affecting the life space.

When conducting family treatment or treatment with couples, a separate life space drawing provides an opportunity to conduct some explorations as to the personal view of the life space. Some therapists of couples counseling like to meet with each member of the couple, not only in a combined session but also in individual sessions to investigate more details with each member of the couple. Conducting the FLSD with an individual allows for the easy transmission of knowledge about the person while possibly revealing nonverbal messages not previously expressed in conjoint sessions. Comparing individual drawings with the couple's combined drawing facilitates an opportunity to look for congruency and differences.

Developing an individual FLSD was also part of the original model of STMFI (Mostwin, 1980a, p. 64). The individual FLSD provides some individual expression to family therapy treatment by creating an environment and process for clients to share information that they might not have felt safe to provide in the conjoint family session. The individual FLSD is another opportunity for the client to engage in the treatment process by providing another level of nonverbal communication that help to gain insights about the client's experience.

Individual FLSD: Case Example 6.A

The following drawing is from a single, 28-year-old Caucasian woman. Her ethnic background includes European ancestry, and her family has lived in the United States for many generations. She is seeking counseling due to feelings of depression and frustration with her life. She recently broke up with her boyfriend and has some sadness around the breakup. She is living alone and has no pets. Her parents divorced when she was 8 years old and as a child she lived with her mother and various male friends of her mother along with two siblings. Currently her mother has a steady boyfriend. The client is living independently and has viable employment. She was born and raised in the general location that she currently lives in. Her parents are living as well as her grandparents.

Steps Three and Four: Placement of Self and Significant Others

Key to Drawing Step 3 and 4: Placement of Self and Significant Others

Me: client
M: mother
MB: mother's boyfriend
F: father
FGF: father's girlfriend
S: sister
B: brother

OB: her old boyfriend
MGM: maternal grandmother
MGF: maternal grandfather
PGM: paternal grandmother
PGF: paternal grandfather
A: aunt
U: uncle

Placement of Self

The client places herself at the top of the drawing in the outer zone at the 12:00 position of the control circle. This position does suggest some authority and confidence, according to Mostwin (1980a).

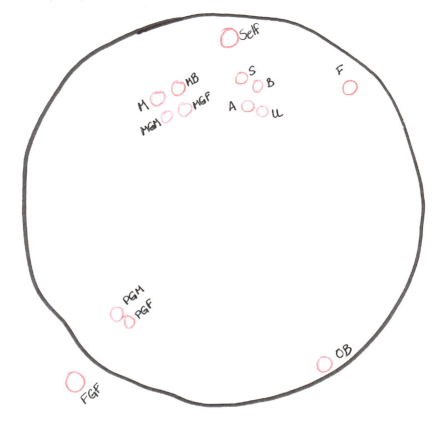

Figure 6.1 Steps three and four: placement of self and significant others, Example 6.A

Table 6.1 Steps three and four: zone, region, placement, and size, Example 6.A

Individual drawing example 1
Outside: father's girlfriend 7:00
Outer: client 12:00, father 2:00, old boyfriend 5:00, paternal grandfather and grandmother 7:00 partial
Middle: mother 11:00, mother's boyfriend 11:00, maternal grandmother 11:00, maternal grandfather 11:00, aunt 12:00, uncle 1:00, brother 12:00, sister 12:00
Inner: no symbols
Size: all symbols are similar and on the small side

Significant Others

The mother of the client is located just on the edge between the middle zone, edging close to the outer zone in the 11:00 position on the left side of the drawing. Next to her in this same zone is her current boyfriend. Below the symbol for the mother are located the maternal grandparents, also in the middle zone getting closer to the 11:00 position. Getting close to the center zone and located just above it near the 12:00 are the maternal aunt and her husband. The father is located in the 2:00 position in the outer zone of the drawing. The old boyfriend is located in the outer circle in the 5:00 position. Also located in the lower half of the FLSD are her paternal grandparents located near the 7:00 region.

Size

The symbols for people including herself would be considered on the small size of what we normally see in the drawings.

The client's closest symbols are for her sister at 1.5 cm and her brother at 2 cm. The symbols at the greatest distance from her symbol are Father's girlfriend at 16.5 cm and her old boyfriend at 15 cm away from her symbol.

Table 6.2 Step four, significant others: distance from symbol for self, Example 6.A

Mother	3.5 cm
Mother's boyfriend	2.5 cm
Father	5 cm
Father's girlfriend	16.5 cm
Aunt	2.5 cm
Uncle	3 cm
Sister	1.5 cm
Brother	2 cm
Old boyfriend	15 cm
Maternal grandmother	4 cm
Maternal grandfather	3.5 cm
Paternal grandmother	13 cm
Paternal grandfather	13.5 cm

Reflections on Steps Three and Four: Individual Case Example 6.A

This drawing does not have any people in the emotional center of the drawing. This representation is not unusual for single people living on their own, but it needs to be explored with the client to determine the client's sense of family. Her sense of self seems strong as reflected in the top position, although it would be worth checking issues around sense of self due to size. The drawing does indicate some isolation from parents, with each one on separate sides. This is also common among people who grew up in homes where the parents were divorced. She also locates symbols for her parents in lower positions, which requires some investigating as to learning more about her experience with parents and her role in the family. This drawing shows a lot of empty space in the middle, and it is important to explore what it is like to have nothing in the middle of the drawing.

STEP FIVE: ENVIRONMENTAL SYMBOLS

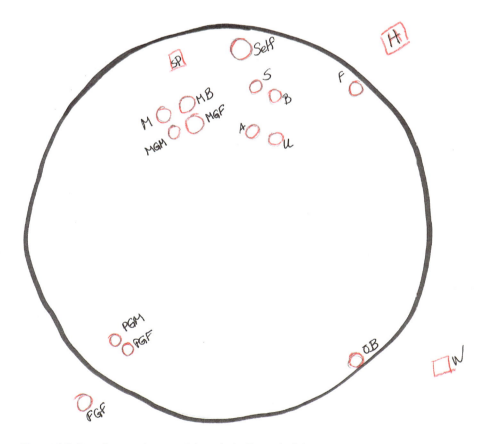

Figure 6.2 Step five: environmental symbols, Example 6.A

Table 6.3 Step five, environmental symbols: zone, region, size, and distance, Example 6.A

Outside: work 5:00, hobby 2:00
Outer: spiritual practice 11:00 and 12:00
Middle: no symbols
Inner: no symbols
Size: similar in size to each other
Distance: work 17 cm, hobby 5.9 cm, spiritual practice 2.7 cm

Key to Symbols

H: hobby   W: work   SP: spiritual practice

Placement

The client placed three symbols for environmental factors. Work was placed outside the circle in the lower section of the drawing near the 5:00 position. The client's hobby was placed in the 2:00 position outside the circle in the upper half of the life space. A symbol for spiritual practice was located between the 11:00 and 12:00 position in the outer zone near the edge of the circle.

Size

The size of these symbols is also considered relatively small for FLSD.

Distance

The symbols for this drawing indicate that most of the environmental symbols are located outside of the family life space. Spiritual practice is located inside the FLSD, 2.7 cm from the client's symbol. The client's hobby is located 5.9 cm away, and the symbol for work is located 17 cm away. Work is the most distant symbol in the whole life space.

Reflections on Step Five: Individual Case Example 6.A

This client has few environmental factors in her life, and those that she does have are located at some distance outside the life space. It would be important to explore her experiences of her job and her hobbies. From this drawing, it would appear that her work is unimportant to her and that she might not like her job. Her symbol for spiritual practice is small but it is located in a powerful position, so it might have some potential as a resource for her. Once again exploring these factors assist the client in determining the focus for counseling efforts.

STEP SIX: STRESS SYMBOLS

The client only indicated one stress in this life space but indicated that the symbol represented her life and everything in her life. She expressed frustration and a sense of being overwhelmed.

USING FLSD WITH DIFFERENT TYPES OF CLIENTS

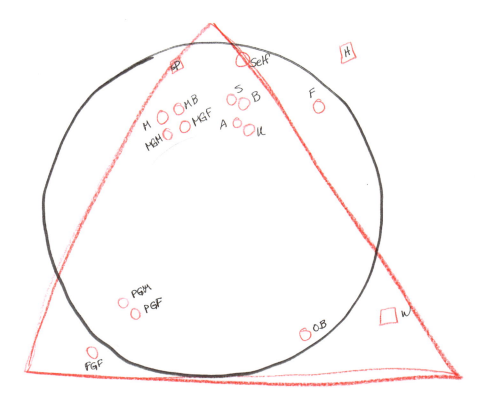

Figure 6.3 Step six: stress symbols, Example 6.A

Placement

The only symbol for this client was placed over her whole life space circle. The symbol includes everything but her symbol for her hobby and her symbol for her father.

Size

The size of this symbol takes up the whole past and is in a remarkable contrast to other symbols in the drawing. The client is letting us know that she has a large stress and that it involves all aspects of her life space. While not uncommon in our observations, the evidence of large symbols reflects an important symbol demonstrating strong feelings in regard to stress. Large symbols often include multiple stresses and indicate a sense of being overwhelmed.

Distance

The symbol for life stress has no distance from the client's personal symbol and engulfs all of the other symbols except for the hobby and the symbol for her father.

Reflections on Step Six: Individual Case Example 6.A

The symbol for stress is one of the most striking aspects of this FLSD. The large triangle covering the whole page stands out especially when viewed with the smaller symbols for people and environmental factors. It would be important to explore the meaning of the stress symbol and identify the component parts of this stress. Noticing that the father's symbol is excluded from the stress symbol provides another opportunity to process the potential meaning of not including this parent in the stress symbol.

USING THE FLSD WITH INDIVIDUAL CASE EXAMPLE 6.A

In developing the treatment plan we processed the FLSD with the client. As we explored the symbols, we discovered that she does have some emotional stress with both her parents and often felt like she was in the middle of her parent's issues. She was asked about what is it like to have such a big space in the center of this drawing, and what was it like to have that large stress symbol over the whole life space. She reflected that it is overwhelming and she wants to have a better control on the circumstances of her life. She did comment that she often felt like she did not have one family but two. At the point of creating the drawing, she feels like she has some management of the issue with her parents but does not like her father's current girlfriend. She senses that her father's current girlfriend does not like her and resents any time that the father spends with her. The client often feels that the father would choose his girlfriend over her if there was a choice between attending to one or the other. Her main attachment concern is that she does not feel that others think that her needs are important, but that she must take care of others to have value.

The client's intention for therapy and treatment was to process her relationship struggles with her ex-boyfriend. We counseled her from an attachment theory framework. She was able to look at her family of origin experiences and see where she experienced her partner as distant in a similar way that she experienced her mother and father both choosing others over her needs. She was able to develop a sense of how she would conduct relationship interactions in a new manner when developing new romantic partners. She was able to explore how her attachment injury related to overcompensating and putting her needs aside to be a caretaker allowed her to maintain situations such as unpleasant work environments without a proper set of boundaries.

INDIVIDUAL FLSD: CASE EXAMPLE 6.B

This example demonstrates a drawing from a married 40-year-old African American male (many generations having lived in the United States). He is married for the second time and has one child, aged 10, from this current relationship and no other children. His mother died when he was a child and he did not have contact with her parents, who also died when he was young. He has little information about his mother's side of the family. His father remarried and he has two siblings from his father's second marriage. This client is a college graduate working in the technology field. He was raised in another locality and state and his parents recently relocated to be near him. His wife's family also lives nearby. She has living parents and one brother. He is currently requesting relationship counseling. This is an example of a drawing with one person and not the couple.

Steps Three and Four: Placement of Self, Significant Others

Key to Symbols

S: self	MGM: maternal grandmother
W: wife	MGF: maternal grandfather
So: Son	WF: wife's father
F: father	WM: wife's mother
M: mother	Si: sister
SM: stepmother	B: brother
PGF: paternal grandfather	BIL: brother-in-law
PGM: paternal grandmother	Dog: pet

Placement of Self

The client placed himself in the center of the circle. The center of the control circle indicates emotional connection to the family (Mostwin, 1980b).

Significant Others

The client placed his wife intersecting with his symbol in the center of the drawing also located in the emotional center. The client has most of his other family members near the emotional center. He has placed his paternal grandparents at the top of his symbol in the emotional center. He has placed his son connecting to his circle just at his left. He has placed his father slightly below him. The symbol for his wife's father is also located just below his father's symbol getting close to the middle zone location. Continuing around the inner circle to the right, we see his symbol for his brother also intersecting his own symbol, located in the inner circle. To the right of his symbol for the brother, he places a symbol for his sister that intersects the symbol for his wife. Most of the symbols for people intersect in some fashion. Symbols located in the lower half of the drawing are the dogs, and then above the symbol for dogs are his wife's mother and brother-in-law. These symbols are all in the inner zone. Outside of the family life space located in the upper right-hand corner of the drawing are symbols for his mother and his maternal grandparents.

Size

Most of the symbols are good size, indicating strong sense of presence and self. We notice the largest symbols are for himself, his wife, and his father. The smallest symbols are representing his mother and her parents.

Distance

The most remarkable observation we make from this drawing is the closeness of all the symbols and their position in the center. Most of the symbols intersect and connect to each other, so measuring distance is difficult. The symbol for his mother located 11.5 cm from client's symbol is the most distant symbol at we see in the drawing. Located below mother's symbol are the symbols for his maternal grandparents measured at 9.7 cm for his maternal grandfather and 11.5 cm for the maternal grandmother. These symbols stand in stark contrast to all the other symbols that are drawn very close to the center.

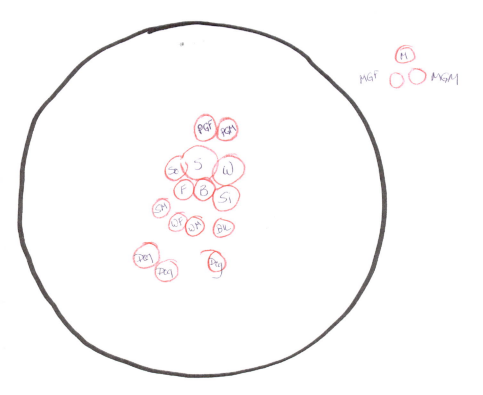

Figure 6.4 Steps three and four: placement of self and significant others, Example 6.B

Table 6.4 Steps three and four, placement of self and significant others: zone, region, size, and distance, Example 6.B

Outside: mother 2:00; maternal grandmother 2:00, maternal grandfather 2:00

Outer: no symbols

Middle: some inner symbols have edges in the middle zone; paternal grandfather and paternal grandmother 12:00, dog 6:00 and 7:00

Inner: self 12:00, wife 12:00, son 1:00, father 9:00, stepmother 9:00, dog 7;00, dog 6:00, dog 6:00, brother-in-law 6:00, sister 3:00, wife's mother 6:00, wife's father 7:00

Size: large symbols; his is the largest with wife, father, and dogs; smallest is MGM and MGF

Distance: wife, father, son, paternal grandfather, paternal grandmother, brother, symbols touch or intersect his symbol, mother 11.5 cm, maternal grandfather 9.7 cm, maternal grandmother 10.3 cm, wife's mother 2.2 cm, brother-in-law 2.5 cm, sister 1 cm, wife's father 1.8, stepmother 2.5, dog 3.7 cm, dog 4 cm, dog 3 cm

Reflections on Steps Three and Four: Individual Case Example 6.B

In viewing this drawing we see that the emotional center of the drawing has most of the relatives and people in his life close to the client. We would observe that the client has an intensity and passion for people in his life and that his family, even in-laws and stepparent relatives, are very important to him and he has a sense of close family connections. This type of closeness can be a strength but also a source of stress.

The important exception to all of the close family member symbols is related to the symbol for his mother and her family who are located outside the circle in the upper right-hand of the page. We note that his mother died when he was very young and that he did not have active memory or a sense of relationship with her or her family. It might be a logical assumption to assume that the mother's placement was due to this lack of actual life connection and his mother's death when he was a child. The location of deceased relatives outside the circle is not unexpected because they died when he was a child. Even though they are outside the family circle, he places them in a position of respect. The mother is located in a powerful position but she is experienced with great emotional distance. It is not uncommon for people to place deceased relatives they never met inside the life space. But in this case, he has placed his mother and her relatives outside the family circle. His experience of his sense of relationship with his mother is worth investigating, and it is something we would follow up on as therapists working with an attachment framework. This would be especially important if it affects his sense of connection to his wife. Therapy models that utilize family of origin frameworks would follow up on this information. Other models might log it as an interesting fact but pursue therapeutic goals connected to their own frameworks, focusing more on problem-solving the client's expressed concerns.

STEP FIVE: ENVIRONMENTAL SYMBOLS

Key to Symbols

HW: work   SS: son's School
H: hobby   WW: wife's work

Placement

Work is placed in the middle zone at the 3:00 zone inside the life space. Wife's work and son's school are located in lower 3:00 positions in the middle zone. The lower outer zone holds the symbol for hobby and is located in the 5:00 zone.

Size

These symbols are smaller than most of the symbols for people in this drawing. The symbol for his work is the largest, followed by his wife's work and then his hobby symbol. His son's school is symbolized by the smallest square symbol in the drawing.

Distance

The symbol for hobby is located 8.3 cm away from his symbol. His wife's work is 5.7 cm away from his symbol and the son's school is 4.2 cm away from his symbol.

THE INDIVIDUAL FAMILY LIFE SPACE DRAWING

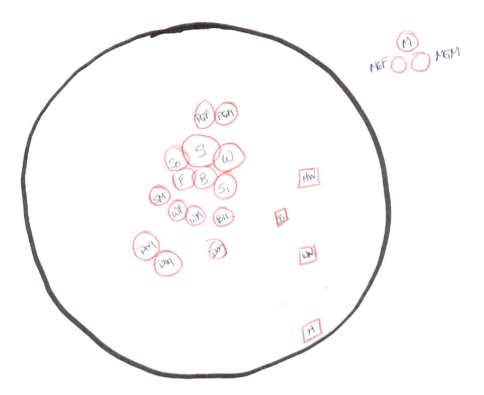

Figure 6.5 Step five: environmental symbols, Example 6.B

Table 6.5 Step five: environmental symbols, Example 6.B

work	zone and region	size	distance
wife's work	Middle zone, 3:00 region	smaller than symbol for self	4.6 cm
	Middle zone, 4:00	similar to other symbols	5.7 cm
hobby	zone and region	size	distance
	outer, 5:00	smaller than self symbol	8.3 cm
son's school	zone and region	size	distance
	inner edge, 3:00	smallest symbol	4.2 cm

Reflections on Step Five: Individual Case Example 6.B

The symbols for environmental and institutional factors in this drawing do not appear to hold the emotional intensity of the people in this life space as reflected by the locations of the symbols. The symbols are not unusually small, but they are smaller than most of the symbols for family members. The hobby symbol is the least important to him. His comments at the time of the drawing indicated that he was not able to pursue these hobbies due to time constraints.

Step Six: Stress Symbols

Key to Symbols

R: relationship issues   WM: wife's mother   H: hobbies

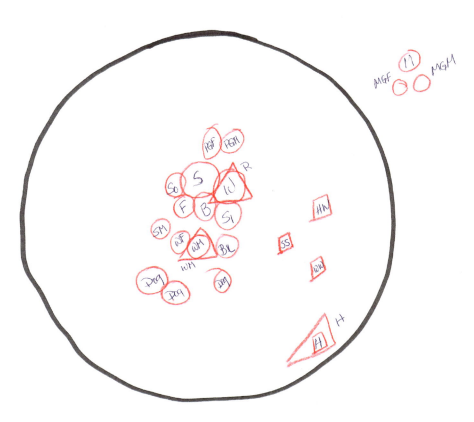

Figure 6.6 Step six: stress symbols, Example 6.B

Table 6.6 Step six, stress symbols: zone, region, size, and distance, Example 6.B

relationship	zone and region inner 12:00	size large similar to other	distance no distance
wife's mother	zone and region inner 6:00	size large, similar to other symbols	distance 1.5 cm
hobbies	zone and region outer 5:00	size large, similar to others	distance 7.5 cm

THE INDIVIDUAL FAMILY LIFE SPACE DRAWING

Placement

The symbol for relationship issues is located in the center zone over the symbols for the client's wife. The symbol for stress related to his mother-in-law is located between the center zone directly over the symbol for the mother-in-law. The stress symbol for hobbies is located in the lower outer zone directly over the environmental symbol for hobbies.

Size

The size of these symbols is large enough to indicate a strong sense of stress over the situation. The symbol size is in keeping with the other symbols drawn in the life space and indicate some intensity and concern related to the issue. The symbol size is about the same for each symbol, 2 cm to 2.5 cm in size.

Distance

The symbol for stress related to his wife is the closest symbol to him, with actually no space between the stress symbol and his own symbol. The stress symbol for wife's mother is 2 cm. The last stress symbol for hobby is about 7.5 cm from the client's symbol for himself.

Reflections on Step Six: Individual Case Example 6.B

The most dramatic stress symbol we see in this drawing relates to his relationship with his wife and his mother-in-law. The whole drawing reflects close family connections and it is a natural consequence that problems within the family center are most likely to facilitate increased anxiety and stress for his life. We see the stress as a sign that his marriage is important to him and that he is invested in working on the issues that are problematic at this time. The hobby stress, while significant in size, balances out with the location in the lower outer zone. That indicates less significance. A stress and environmental factor related to hobbies does not reflect a concern but might be a contributing factor to other stresses in the life space. This stress symbol is a hint as to potential therapeutic paths to investigate in the course of therapy.

STEP EIGHT: COMMUNICATION LINES: INDIVIDUAL CASE EXAMPLE 6.B

This client completed communication lines on separate sheet of paper with the therapist. The lines to people revealed:

    Good to son

    Good to father

    Good to wife

    Good to wife's father

    So-so to wife's mother

    Good to brother

    Good and sometimes so-so to sister

    Good to wife's brother

    Good to paternal grandmother

So-so to paternal grandfather

Poor to mother

Poor to maternal grandparents

So-so to stepmother

Good to dogs

These communication symbols are positive an in sync with our understanding of the locations and placements of these people in the life space.

Using the FLSD With Individual Case Example 6.B

The goal of completing this life space drawing was to allow an individual in couple's treatment to meet with the therapist and explore issues related to commitment to the relationship and to see if the individual drawing was in sync with the couples drawing. This drawing helps the attachment-based therapist to explore more information about the family of origin and to explore his emotional sense of connection to deceased mother and her family.

This drawing helped the therapist to see that the drawing was in sync with the couples combined FLSD. The man placed himself in similar position in his combined drawing and with the same size of circles along with distances. We see that the client was comfortable in providing information in the couple's sessions in the same way that he did in the individual session. The symbols will help the therapists to explore factors affecting quality of connection in the relationship. An example of using the communication lines to assist with investigating the client situation is to notice something such as the good communication line drawn to the wife but also the large stress symbol placed over the symbol for the wife. Asking questions related to the symbols and lines enables the conversation toward more detailed information.

Individual FLSD: Case Example 6.C

The following example demonstrates something that we rarely see in completing the FLSD. This person decided to complete the drawing with all of the symbols outside the life space. This drawing is an example of the infinite possibilities that can occur as a result of completing the FLSD. The case example is from a 24-year-old Caucasian American heterosexual male of European descent. He is living with his parents, attending school, and working two jobs to support himself. His parents provide some financial support by providing housing and food. He is required to work and pay his school tuition and other expenses after having previously dropping out of college in the past. He has a girlfriend and a network of friends. He is seeking counseling because he wants to be successful in school and work toward becoming independent from his parents.

Steps Three and Four: Placement of Self and Significant Others

Key to Symbols

Me: client   Fr: friend
Mom: mother   GF: girlfriend

THE INDIVIDUAL FAMILY LIFE SPACE DRAWING

F: father
B: brother
BGF: brother's girlfriend
Sis: sister
BF: sister's boyfriend

PGM: paternal grandmother
PGF: paternal grandfather
MGM: maternal grandmother
MGF: paternal grandfather

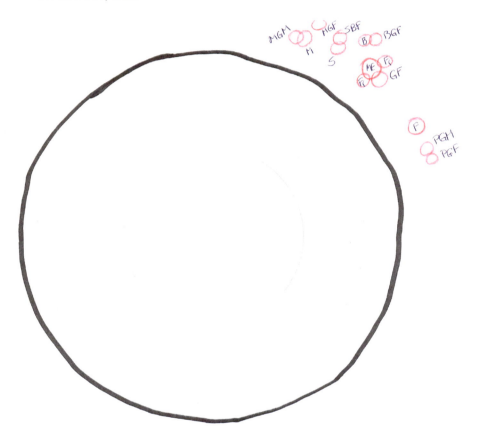

Figure 6.7 Steps three and four: placement of self and significant others, Example 6.C

Table 6.7 Steps three and four: zone, region, size, and distance, Example 6.C

Outside: mom 12:00, dad 2:00, brother 1:00, brother's girlfriend 2:00, sister 1:00, sister's boyfriend 1:00, friend 2:00, girlfriend 1:00, paternal grandmother and paternal grandfather 2:00, maternal grandmother 12:00, maternal grandfather 1:00, self 1:00

Outer: no symbols

Middle: no symbols

Inner: no symbols

Size: small symbols

Table 6.8 Step three, significant others: distance, Example 6.C

client	father	brother	brother's girlfriend	friend	friend	girlfriend
	2.8	1 cm	1 cm	0 cm	0 cm	0 cm
mother	sister	sister's boyfriend	PGM	PGF	MGM	MGF
2.8 cm	1.2 cm		4.2 cm	4.5 cm	3 cm	3 cm

Placement of Self

The client locates himself outside the family life space and begins to create his own separate life space outside the circle. He is located in the upper right-hand corner of the sheet, just above the 1:00 position.

Significant Others

The client places all significant people outside the FLSD symbol. He places his mom above him outside the place of 1:00 along with her parents above her intersecting her placement. The MGF is placed above the MGM and to the right. He places his brother and brother's girlfriend, who intersects brother's symbol, above him. The client's sister outside 1:00 is also located above the client between him and his mother to the left of his symbol. He places the sister's boyfriend intersecting her symbol but in a slightly dominant position. Next to the client, to the right and to the left of his symbol, he places two friends. These friends also intersect his symbol. Below his symbol intersecting his own circle he places a symbol for a girlfriend. He places his father outside the circle near the 2:00 position. Below the father he places his paternal grandparents who also intersect just outside the circle near the 3:00 position.

Size

The symbols are not large and not particularly small in relation to each other and the space on the paper. The smallest circles are for friends, girlfriends, and paternal grandparents.

Distance

The client places himself 11.3 cm from the center of the family life space. The other symbols for family members are located near him. His maternal grandmother is located 3.5 cm from his own symbol. His maternal grandfather is on the other side of his mother at 3 cm away from his symbol. Both symbols for the maternal grandparents are above him and the symbol for his mother. The mother's symbol is 2.8 cm away from his own symbol. His brother is located near him above him, 1 cm away, and his sister slightly more distant to the left at 1.2 cm away.

Around the symbol for himself, he places his symbol for friends intersecting his own symbol, so there is no space between them. He does the same for his girlfriend, who is below him and his friends. Her symbol intersects the client's personal symbol.

Below the symbol for himself, he places his father's symbol at 2.8 cm away. Below the symbol for his father he places his grandparents. The paternal grandmother is 4.2 cm away and the paternal grandfather is 4.5 cm away. The paternal grandparents are the most distant position in his outer circle representation.

Reflections on Steps Three and Four: Individual Case Example 6.C

When viewing this picture, it appears that the client decided to create an alternate life space outside the lines of the family circle. We could detect a creative attempt to design a family outside traditional concepts as he develops his own separate life space in the upper right-hand corner of the page. This conception might be surmised in seeing family members close to his own symbol. We could deduce that he is attempting to individuate and develop his own new life space as he separates from his own family of origin. There is some concern from us, the authors, as we observe this FLSD by noting that no family member is located in the center. It could reflect problems within the family and a lost sense of what family is supposed to be. The parents might be considering an end to their marital relationship and the family could be reforming. There is some suspicion that family has not always been a "happy or good" concept for this person by drawing everyone outside the life space. It is a piece of information that needs to be investigated in the course of counseling. His relationships with friends has lasted longer than his relationship with his girlfriend, which might be reflected in the placements of friends beside him and the girlfriend below him. We do observe some strengths with close relationships of siblings and friends, even with the presence of intersecting circles, which often indicate some lack of differentiation.

STEP FIVE: ENVIRONMENTAL SYMBOLS

Key to Symbols

   R: relationship
   S: school
   GW: girlfriend's work
   NJ: new job
   OJ: old job

Placement

Once again, all of the environmental symbols are located on the outside of the symbol for the family life space. He places the symbol for his relationship with his girlfriend below him outside the 2:00 position. He places a symbol to his right slightly below him for school, and he places a symbol for a new job on the other side of him. On the opposite side and corner of the paper containing the FLSD, the client has placed a symbol for his old job diagonal to his own position outside the 7:00 position on the control circle.

Size

The size of these symbols in relation to other symbols show the largest symbol to be his relationship with girlfriend. The symbol for work is middle size and the symbol for school new job and girlfriend's work are all relatively the same. The size of the symbol for the old job is one of his largest symbols. The location of the symbol is distant from the rest of the symbols, but the size of the symbol might indicate some emotional attachment.

Distance

The symbols for environmental factors also show a symbolic representation of closeness with one exception. The symbol for his old job is located 23 cm away from his own symbol

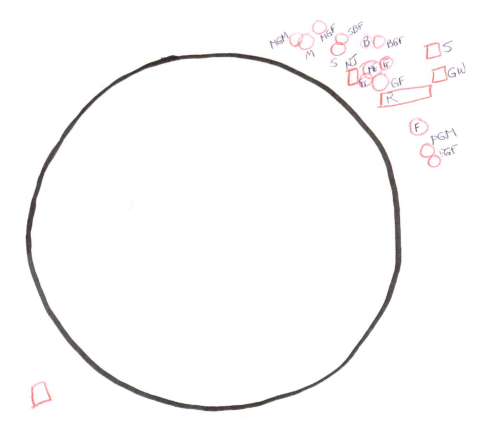

Figure 6.8 Step five: environmental symbols, Example 6.C

Table 6.9 Step five, environmental symbols: zone, region, size, and distance, Example 6.C

Symbol	Zone and region	Size	Distance
School	Outside 1:00	Small	2 cm
Girlfriend's work	Outside 1:00	Small	1.8 cm
New job	Outside 1:00	Small	.2 cm
Old job	Outside 7:00	Larger than others	23 cm
Relationship	Outside 2:00	Long rectangle larger	1 cm

outside the life space. Other symbols for relationship measure 1 cm from his own symbol, and his new job is 0.2 cm from his own symbol. His school is 2 cm away from his symbol, and his girlfriend's work is 1.8 cm away from his symbol. Most of these symbols would be considered very close to him.

THE INDIVIDUAL FAMILY LIFE SPACE DRAWING | 91

Reflections on Step Five: Individual Case Example 6.C

The environmental symbol has stayed with the client in his own life space outside the family life space and are significant and close to him with the exception of his symbol for work. His symbol for his old job represents a menial job that he does not like and only participates in because he is need of the money. He lets us know that he has worked there many years but feels mistreated and taken advantage of by his superiors. His new job is more exciting because it is connected to his future career vision. From the placement and size of the symbol for his girlfriend, we see that his relationship with the girlfriend is very important to him.

STEP SIX: STRESS SYMBOLS

Key to Symbols

M: mom F: father
NW: new job OJ: old job
R: relationship

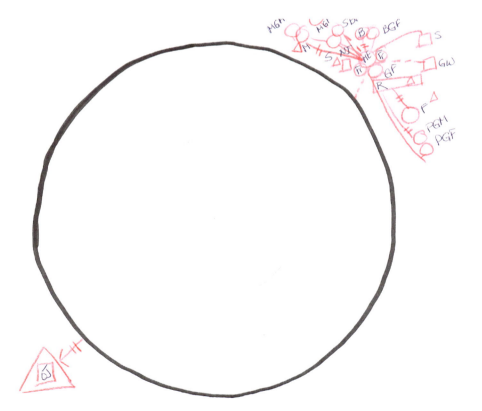

Figure 6.9 Steps six and eight: stress symbols and communication lines, Example 6.C

Table 6.10 Step six, stress symbols: zone, region, size, and distance, Example 6.C

Stress	Zone and region	Size	Distance
Mom	Outside 12:00	small	2.9 cm
New job	Outside 1:00	small	1 cm
Relationship	Outside 2:00	small	2 cm
Father	Outside 2:00	small	3 cm
Old job	Outside 7:00	Large	22.7 cm

Placement

Stress symbols are drawn near the person or environmental factor symbolically represented in the life space. In this instance, the client placed a stress symbol near his mother located outside the 12:00 position and near grandparents but indicates it is about his mother. He placed a stress symbol within the symbol for time with his girlfriend at the lower right inside that symbol. That symbol was located between the 1:00 and 2:00 position. There is also a stress symbol for his relationship with his dad just above the 3:00 position stress symbol, just above the symbol for his dad. Just above the environmental symbol for the new job in the upper left-hand corner of that symbol. All of the stress symbols are again located close to his outside grouping of his own family life space. There is one exception, as we have previously observed, with the symbol for his old job. This symbol is located in the lower left corner of the drawing page just outside the 7:00 position.

Size

All of the symbols for stress in this drawing are particularly small, with the exception of the old job work stress. The work stress symbol located in the lower outside corner is relatively large in comparison to all the symbols previously drawn in the life space. The stresses located near him and his significant others are small in relation to the other symbols they are connected to.

Distance

The stress symbols are placed close to the people and places they symbolize. The stress related to work is 22.7 cm away from his own symbol. Closer to him is the symbol for the new job, 1 cm. His stress for his time with his girlfriend is 2 cm. The relationship with parent stress is 2.9 cm for his mother and 3 cm with his father.

Reflections on Step Six: Individual Case Example 6.C

The stress symbols reveal that he has some conflict with his parents but that the stresses do not seem major. He does reflect while conducting this process that he has often felt in the middle of his parents, as the drawing reflects. He tells the counselor that his parents fight and he does not like to get in the middle of their arguments. He also indicates that they are pressing him to get on with his life and they hassle him about his decisions and life plans. His stress symbols do not seem overwhelming in this drawing, with the exception of his old job work stress symbol. He does not like this job and is looking forward to the time when he can leave this place of employment to a better paying job and career.

Step Eight: Communication Lines

Key to Symbols

Mom: so-So, sometimes good
Father: poor
Brother: poor
Sister: good
Girlfriend: good
Friends: good
Maternal grandmother: poor
Maternal grandfather: so-so
Paternal grandfather: poor
Paternal grandmother: poor

New job: good
School: good
Girlfriend's work: so-so
Relationship: good
My work: so-so

Stress to Mom: so-so
Stress to Dad: poor
Stress to old job: poor

Reflections on Step Eight: Individual Case Example 6.C

These lines indicate some consistency with symbol placements. The closest symbols have good communication lines and distant ones have poor communication lines, with the exception of his work. Work is given a so-so line above the large circle but the stress symbol is given a poor communication line. We see some so-so lines to his relationship with his mother and his maternal grandfather and a poor communication line to his maternal grandmother. Girlfriend's work is so-so for him because he does not like the hours she has to work, which conflict with his time off.

Using the FLSD With Individual Case Example 6.C

The plan for counseling intends to explores his desire to individuate and work toward independence. Cognitive behavioral approaches could focus on desired outcomes and behaviors that enhance or impair the desired outcomes. Emotional explorations could define attitudes and self-defeating feelings that compromise the obtainment of his goals.

Family of origin therapists could explore his anxiety around his parents' marriage and his sense of being in the middle to help him separate his emotional expressions from the behavior of his parents. There are many ways to approach this presentation in the FLSD. Strengths-based approaches would focus on his strong sense of self as he takes his family outside of the life space to create something new.

Summary: Individual Family Life Space Drawing

The individual life space is the process where a client can report their sense of self and significant family members without the influences of others in the life space. It is not unusual to see different placements when individual complete the drawing without other family members nearby. Taking time to complete the FLSD with individuals allows for the perspective of the individual person and sometimes can reveal intentions for desired placements. Sometimes people will indicate that while their family member sees them in a specific location, they will voice the concern that they see themselves in another location. Or they may express an observation such as "my family sees me here, but I want to be in this position." In any event, the individual drawing is a process to explore family relationships and sense of self that might not be spoken but symbolically portrayed in the process of the drawing.

REFERENCES

Mostwin, D. (1980a). *Social dimension of family treatment*. Washington, DC: National Association of Social Workers.

Mostwin, D. (1980b). Life space approach to the study and treatment of a family. In D. Mostwin (Ed.), *Life space approach to the study and treatment of a family*. Washington, DC: The Catholic University of America.

CHAPTER SEVEN
Family Life Space Drawing: Examples With Couples

FLSD With Couples

The FLSD is an excellent way to conduct an initial session with clients who are seeking marriage or relationship counseling. Meeting both members of the couple in the first session through the process of the FLSD facilitates the therapist in sharing equal time with the couple as they all begin to engage in the treatment process. The therapist/counselor can meet and develop connections with each member of the couple as individuals but view the interplay of the combined life space.

The completed picture of the life space drawings can take on many configurations. Couples can create a drawing that shows family members all over the drawing, or they often create a picture of one color on one side and the partner has space for themselves in another section of the drawing. The final drawing presents an overall picture of how the couple functions together and has combined their lives together.

The FLSD facilitates sharing of information related to relationship crisis and illustrates the situation of a couple undergoing stress due to life cycle changes. We can see areas where the couple agrees or we can see areas of disagreements. The drawing often illustrates areas of concern that might not be typically voiced in first sessions.

The following examples of couple's drawings will illustrate a lesbian couple struggling with relationship stress, a couple navigating transitions to parenthood with a new baby, and an unmarried couple who are evaluating relationship commitments and future decisions about building a life together after the birth of a child. These drawings are but a sample of the possible configurations we can see in creating these drawings. These examples are composites of cases from our experience and are not actual drawings of any specific client.

Couple Case Example 7.A

The following case example demonstrates a FLSD with an unmarried lesbian couple. One member of the couple is a Caucasian American of European descent, 35 years old. The other partner is a Caucasian American of Italian descent, 45 years old. The couple have been in a relationship for 5 years and live together. Neither one of the partners has children. They have contemplated marriage but have delayed that commitment due to some issues with heated arguments and verbal abuse in their relationship. They are seeking relationship counseling to see if they are able to improve their connection and seek ways to communicate without arguing. Both have been involved with individual counseling and now seek relationship counseling together.

Partner One has living parents who have been married over 50 years and live some distance away from the couple. Partner Two has other family members that include a married younger sister who lives with her husband and grown children. These family members also live several states away from the couple. Partner One shares that her childhood was very happy and that parents were supportive. She grew up with a strong sense of her ethnicity as Italian and expresses pride in that nationality. The family professes a Jewish faith that was observed during holidays. Partner One has her own successful business selling real estate.

Partner Two has parents who are currently divorced. Her childhood was difficult and her parents followed an ultra-conservative Christian religion that lived in a tight-knit community. She describes her childhood as abusive emotionally and physically. She has many siblings, including a teenage brother who lives with their mother. Partner Two's mother and some siblings live in a region close to the couple. Partner Two's father is not in a relationship with the family and his whereabouts are unknown. Partner Two does not work outside the home and manages the couple's side business of raising and selling exotic birds. Partner Two reports a history of past suicidal and substance abuse behavior but states that this behavior is not currently present in her life.

Step Three: Placement of Self

P1: red   P2: Green

In step three, each partner places a symbol of a circle on the drawing to indicate where they see themselves in the symbolic drawing of their combined families. The following chart lists the placement zone for each partner's symbol and provides an observation on symbol size.

Reflections on Step Three: Couple Case Example 7.A

The first observation related to the symbol placements indicate that the partners are experiencing a sense of distance between their positions. Partner Two is in an upper position, which represents control and power. This in-and-out symbol placement can represent that the person does not feel all together in the family system or has some ambivalence about whether or not they belong in the family symbol. Partner One is in a lower position, which usually indicates a sense of low self-esteem or a sense of powerlessness and rejection. Partners who represent their symbols in this way are often illustrating the distance and distress experienced in the connection of the relationship.

Step Four: Placing Significant Others

After the partners place their individual symbols, the one at the board is asked to place significant other family members who are not currently in the room. The therapist/facilitator will ask about placing children, parents, other family members, and pets in relation to the family drawing. In this example, the couple does not have children but places extended family members and their pet birds.

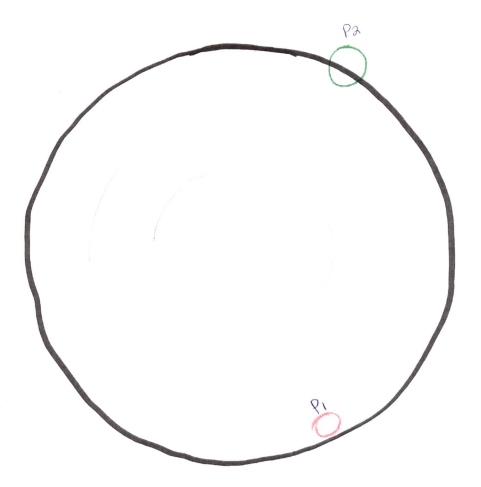

Figure 7.1 Step three, placing individual symbol: couple case, Example 7.A

Table 7.1 Step three: placement of self, Example 7.A

Partner one: red	Partner two: green
Zone and region location: between 6:00 and 7:00 in the outer zone	**Zone and region location:** between the outer zone and outside the family symbol at the 1:00 region
Size of symbol: the symbol size is average	**Size of symbol:** the symbol size is average

Key to Symbols

Partner 1

P1: self	B1: bird 1
Dad: father	B2: bird 2
Mom: mother	B3: bird 3
Sister: sister	B4: bird 4
C1: sister's child	B5: bird 5
C2: sister's child	

Partner 2

M: mother	S6: sibling 6
F: father	S7: sibling 7
S1: sibling 1	B2: bird 2
S2: sibling 2	B3: bird 3
S3: sibling 3	S4: sibling 4

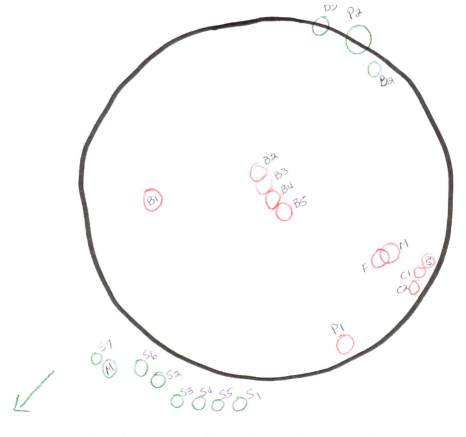

Figure 7.2 Step four, placement of significant others: couple case, Example 7.A

Table 7.2 Step four, significant others: region and zone placements, Example 7.A

Partner one: red	Partner two: green
Outside: no symbols	**Outside:** mother 7:00 region, father extended 7:00 S2 7:00, S3 6:00, S4 6:00, S5 6:00, S1 6:00 B3 partial outside 1:00
Outer: sister 4:00 just above 5:00 C1 and C2, just below her mother, partially located on edge middle zone at 4:00	**Outer:** bird3 partially in 1:00 bird2 2:00
Middle: dad 4:00, partial mother 4:00	**Middle:** no symbols
Inner: bird2 3:00, bird3 3:00, bird4 3:00, bird5 3:00 edging 4:00	**Inner:** no symbols

Table 7.3 Step four, significant others: size and distance, Example 7.A

Partner one: red	Partner two: green
Size: symbols are similar in size to each other	**Size:** symbols are smaller than symbol for self. Family of origin symbols extra small
Distance: dad 2.5 cm, mom 3 cm, sister 4 cm, C1 4 cm, C2 3.7 cm bird1 10.5 cm, bird2 8 cm, bird3 7.5 cm, bird4 6.5 cm, bird5 5.5 cm	**Distance:** mother 20.5 cm, father infinity, S7 20.5 cm, C 20 cm, S5 20.5 cm, S4 20.8, S3 21 cm bird2 1.5 cm, bird3 1.1 cm

Reflections on Step Four: Couple Case Example 7.A

Partner One has family members in the lower section of the drawing, indicating low self-esteem and a sense of powerlessness in family connections. Partner One has parents above their own symbol but close to their own symbol in the lower region joining Partner Two in the powerless position. Partner Two has her family of origin located outside the family symbol with the symbol for her father off the page. Partner Two shares that her family was abusive and that she does not have much contact with this family due to experiencing them as emotionally unsafe. Partner Two does have contact with this family but states that it often does not go well when they are in contact. The size of symbols and placement of Partner Two's family indicate that they are viewed in low regard in a low power position.

The exotic birds in this drawing may represent a sense of emotional support for Partner One. The location of the birds in the inner zone reflect emotional connection and in many instances safety and love. The distance measure from Partner One to the birds is greater than any of her other symbols, but placement in the inner zone counters the distance measure to indicate that the birds are close to the heart of this family. Partner Two places the birds she is closest to near her in the drawing and indicates with her placements that the birds are "her birds." The birds in Partner Two's placement indicate that these particular birds as significant and in high regard for Partner Two. Partner Two did not place all of the birds owned by this couple in the drawing and indicated that she is close to the birds she represented. In this drawing, Bird2 is the only symbol that Partner Two places inside the family symbol. This drawing informs that the birds are very important to this couple.

Step Five: Environmental Symbols

Key to Symbols

Partner One	Partner Two
W: work (bird business)	W: work

Table 7.4 Step five, environmental symbols: zone, region, size, and distance, Example 7.A

Partner one: red	Partner two: green
Outside symbol	Outside symbol
Bird business: covers all regions	Work: partial outside 12:00
Outer zone	Outer zone
Work: 8:00 partial	Work: partial outside 12:00
Middle zone	Middle zone: no symbols
Work: 8:00 partial	
Inner zone: no symbols	Inner zone: no symbols
Size: work size is somewhat large; the symbol for bird business is extra large	Size: similar to symbol for self
Distance: work 6.5 cm, bird business is as close as 1.5 cm and as far as 19.5 cm away	Distance: work 2.5 cm

Reflections on Step Five: Couple Case Example 7.A

This couple does not have many environmental symbols, but the extra-large symbol drawn by Partner One illustrates that the business of the birds takes up a lot emotional energy and time for the couple. Both partners drew symbols related to work. The drawing indicates that work is the primary focus of life for this couple.

Partner One drew her real estate employment as lower in regard than the business of the exotic birds. Partner Two placed work in a high position and shows it as inside and outside the relationship. This visual demonstration conveys that work and the bird business is an important topic to pursue with this couple. Questioning can help process the actual impact of work on this couple. Partner Two does not have employment outside the home business and reflects the significance of her work with the birds by the placement of this symbol in the 12:00 region.

FLSD: EXAMPLES WITH COUPLES | 101

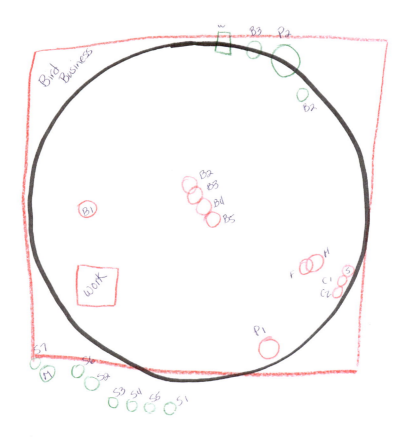

Figure 7.3 Step five, environmental symbols: couple case, Example 7.A

Step Six: Stress Symbols, Example 7.A

Key to Symbols

    Partner 1   **Partner 2**

    R: relationship   Life

Reflections on Step Six: Couple Case Example 7.A

Partner One has one symbol for stress and it is located near the 3:00 position straddling the symbol for family and the world outside the family. The symbol is the only one placed in the drawing. It is the closest symbol to Partner Two, In the drawing and indicates relationship stress. The symbol is large enough to indicate that it is a significant stress to Partner One. The size of the relationship symbol compared to the symbol for the self represents a larger symbol.

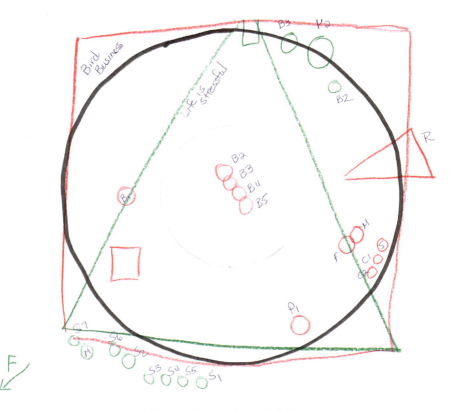

Figure 7.4 Step six, stress symbols: couple case, Example 7.A

Table 7.5 Step six, stress symbols: zone, region, size, and distance, Example 7.A

Partner one: red, relationship stress	Partner two: green, life stress
Placement: outside zone and outer zone 3:00 region	Placement: outside zone, encompassing all the regions of the control circle
Size: large symbol	Size: large symbol
Distance: 9 cm from own symbol	Distance: as close as 2 cm and as distant as 22.5 cm

The position of this one and only drawn stress partially outside the family symbol may indicate that Partner One is somewhat ambivalent about the relationship. The symbol is of significant size and it is on the level of the inner part of the control center and near the heart of the family. The relationship is important but the symbol placement indicates some difficulty for the couple.

There is only one stress symbol for Partner Two in this drawing, but it takes up the whole symbol for the family in this drawing. Partner Two expresses a sense of being overwhelmed with the difficulties of managing the birds and the business related to them. The stress symbol engulfs the center of the family symbol, including the birds and Partner One and her family and work. The size of this symbol is significant, and we get a strong idea about the nature of this stress in the life of this couple as seen by Partner Two. Symbols of this size are indicators of the magnitude of stress levels, and in this situation we can see that the stress level for Partner Two is very high. The large stress symbol in this drawing does not include Partner Two and her birds. It is possible that Partner Two sees the source of stress outside of herself and residing with the partner and the partner's activities. In this situation, it would be useful to explore more details about the specific stresses affecting Partner Two that are component parts of the symbol represented. These types of large symbols are indications for asking more questions and validating the person as part of the engagement process.

STEP EIGHT: COMMUNICATION LINES

Key to Symbols

Partner One:

Mother: good
Father: good
Sister: so-So
Niece: so-So
Nephew: so-so
Bird1: so-so
Bird2: good
Bird3: so-so
Bird4 good
Bird5: good
Work: good
Relationship:so-so
Bird business: so-so

Partner Two

Mother: so-so
Father: poor
Sibling1: poor
Sibling2: so-so
Sibling 3: so-so
Sibling4: poor
Sibling6: poor
Sibling7: good
Bird2: good
Bird3: good
Work: so-so
Stress: poor

Reflections on Step Eight: Couple Case Example 7.A

Exploring the concept of the communication lines allows the facilitator/therapist to see congruencies with positions of symbols and the identification of good, so-so, or poor communication lines. Usually placements outside the family circle will result in so-so or poor communication lines. With this couple, the outside placements are identified with poor and so-so communication lines. Despite the large and significant placements of the business with the birds both partners indicate a so-so relationship with the bird business.

Using the FLSD With Couple Case Example 7.A

This couple has provided a lot of information about underlying emotions in the course of completing this drawing. The drawing was a vehicle for examining the relationship between the couple and investigating the ambivalence that both had toward not only the romantic relationship but also the professional relationship connected to raising and selling exotic birds. The drawing heightened the discussion about current unhappiness and verbal abuse that was ongoing in the relationship.

Even though Partner One was the primary wage earner in the relationship, she describes feelings of failure and distress because no matter what happened, it was difficult to please

Partner Two. Noticing the low position of Partner One in the drawing allowed the therapist to inquire about feelings connected to that position. What is it like being in this position? Exploring the position of Partner Two was useful in eliciting information concerning feelings to being half in and half out of the relationship. Questions related to the position of Partner Two's parents helped initiate conversations about having difficulties trusting love relationships because family members had been a great disappointment in the past.

This couple needs to explore their own ambivalence and stress in this relationship and work on the patterns that get in the way of connection. The relationship already shows some distressful patterns that need to be corrected. Therapy can help guide this couple in working to reverse these patterns or make decisions about boundaries they need to set with each other. The information obtained while in the process of conducting the FLSD revealed more than just background facts; it also opened up emotional content. The drawing reveals and reflects possible difficulties in restoring connection but also reveals insight about the complications of this couple's connections.

Couple Case Example 7.B

The following FLSD demonstrates a middle-class couple seeking marriage counseling after the birth of their first child. This is the first marriage for both members of the couple and they have been in the relationship for 5 years and married for 2 years.

The 30-year-old wife is an Asian American who had been following a career path as a veterinarian. She recently decided to stop working at this profession upon the birth of their son, who is now 4 months old. Her parents are living and married to each other for the last 38 years. She has one sister who is older and married with one child aged 6 years. The parents live about three hours away from the couple's current residence. Her grandparents are deceased. They were the first ones to come to the United States.

The husband in this relationship is a 31-year-old Caucasian American who works at a high-tech job. He also takes care of a farm that the couple owned together, managing a hay business and a few farm goats. His parents are living and live several states away. He has one unmarried sister who lives near the parents. His grandparents are also deceased.

Neither one of the partners has been in counseling before, either individually or as a couple. Neither one reports past experiences with substance abuse or sexual or physical child abuse.

Step Three: Placement of Self

In step three, each member of the couple places a symbol to represent where they see themselves in the family. The following chart provides information concerning zone placement and control circle region as well as comments on size and distance of symbols.

The placements of this couple's symbols indicate some movement of the husband away from the emotional center as he places himself slightly intersecting the middle zone. The wife appears to be in the inner zone but away from the exact center. The husband has a position in the inner zone but slightly off-center. There is some space between the symbols of almost 5 cm; the couple is invested in the family center but appears to have some distance from each other.

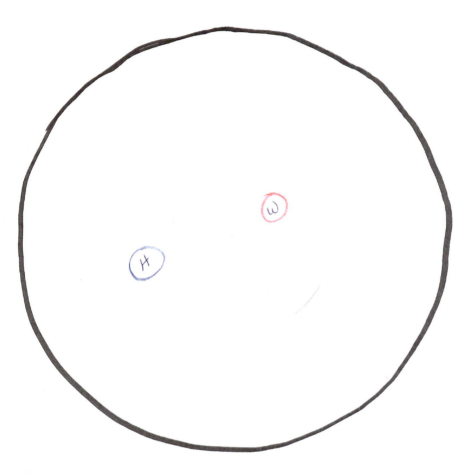

Figure 7.5 Step three, placement of self: couple case, Example 7.B

Table 7.6 Step three: zone, region, placement, size, and distance, Example 7.B

Husband: red	Wife: blue
Location: The husband places himself in the inner zone of the control circle close to the 3:00 region. One section of his symbol is in the middle zone	**Location:** The wife places herself in the inner zone, between 2:00 and 3:00
Size: His symbol size is average size	**Size:** Symbol size average
Distance: His symbol is on the edge of the emotional center of the family	**Distance:** In the emotional center, slightly off-center

Step Four: Placement of Significant Others

After the second member of the couple has placed their symbol for self on the drawing board, that person is asked to place other significant family members, such as children and parents and people who feel like family. In this example, the couple had one child and some extended family members.

Key to Symbols (Wife)

W: wife	N: niece (sister's 6-year-old child)
Son: 4-month-old baby	D: dog
F: father	PGF: paternal grandfather
M: mother	PGM: paternal grandmother
Si: sister	MGF: maternal grandfather
BIL: brother-in-law	MGM: maternal grandmother

Key to Symbols (Husband)

H: husband	MGM: maternal grandmother
Son: 4-month-old baby	MGF: maternal grandfather
M: mother	PGF: paternal grandfather
F: father	PGM: paternal grandmother
Si: sister	U: paternal uncle
D: dog	

Reflections on Step Four: Couple Case Example 7.B

The placements of the wife's family members show the parents and grandparents located in positions above the wife indicating a position of respect and power. The location of some of the grandparents in the outer zone can be reflective of the fact that the grandparents are deceased. We find that people can have an emotional sense of a relative even if the relative is deceased as in the case of this drawing. It is always a good path to pursue when working with this drawing to ask about family traditions and expectations of parental hierarchy according to the origins of family ethnicity and culture. These cultural influences make a difference when understanding the positions of the family drawing. The middle zone holds the majority of the wife's significant other placements, which include her sister paternal grandfather, brother-in-law, and niece. Please note that the niece and brother in-law are partially in the outer zone.

The inner zone of the drawing holds the wife and the 4-month-old son. The family pet is also located near the center of the inner section of the circle in the 5:00 position. The wife also places her parents above her, close to the 12:00 position. The inner zone placements usually represent emotional connections. These family positions reflect traditional hierarchy placements with parents placed in upper positions not too far from her own position. The symbol for the sister is placed to the right of the wife near the 3:00 region. The wife's niece is also in the middle zone near the 3:00 region straddling the edge of that zone and the outer zone. The niece is in a traditional hierarchy placement below her parents. The wife's closest relationships are with her parents, sister, and baby. The greatest distance between any of her symbols in the drawing is between the wife and husband.

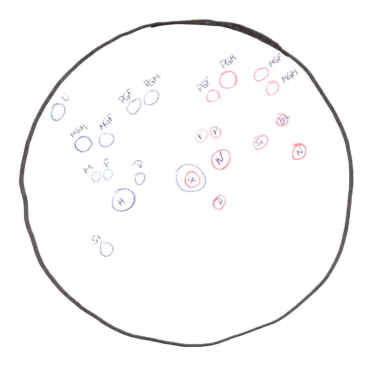

Figure 7.6 Step four, placement of significant others: couple case, Example 7.B.

Table 7.7 Step four, significant others: zone, region, placement, size, and distance, Example 7.B

Husband	Wife
Outside: no symbols	**Outside:** no symbols
Outer: uncle 10:00, partial MGM 10:00	**Outer:** MGF 1:00, MGM 1:00, BIL 2:00, N lower 3:00, partial PGM 12:00
Middle: MGF 10:00, MGM, PGF, PGM 10:00, mother 9:00, father 9:00, sister 8:00, husband partial at 9:00	**Middle:** PGF 12:00, sister 3:00
Inner: husband 9:00, D 9:00, son center	**Inner:** father 12:00, mother 12:00, son center, dog 5:00
Size: symbols are average to small; symbol for son is the largest	**Size:** symbols are similar to each other
Distance: son 2.5 cm, mother 1.5 cm, father 1.3 cm, sister 2 cm, MGM 3.2, MGF 3 cm, PGF 4.8 cm, PGM 5.2 cm uncle 4.8 cm, dog 0.8 cm	**Distance:** son 1.3 cm, mother 1 cm, father 0.8 cm, dog 2 cm sister 1.3 cm, BIL 3.2 cm, N 3.6 cm, MGM 4 cm, MGF 4.5 cm, PGM 4 cm, PGF 3.2 cm

The husband also places the 4-month-old son in the inner zone center and he circled the symbol drawn by his wife, stating that he agreed with his wife that the baby belonged in that spot. Just above the symbol for himself, he places the family dog who also is placed in the inner zone of the family drawing. The husband places himself in the inner zone but with a part of him located in the middle zone to the left of the symbol toward 9:00.

The husband's parents are in the middle zone also near the 9:00 position just above his own symbol. The younger sister is placed to the left of the husband slightly below him, closer to the 8:00 region of the circle. The paternal grandparents are located in the middle zone of the circle above the husband closer to the 11:00 region of the family symbol. The maternal grandfather is located in the middle zone near the 10:00 region. The husband placed a symbol for his paternal uncle in the outer zone just below the 10:00 position. In viewing the placements of the symbols between his symbol and the symbols for family members, we see that most of the symbols are relatively close to his own placement on the left side of the drawing.

The husband's family of origin placements show that he has his family of origin members near him, all close to the 9:00 and 10:00 level of the drawing. The parental placements show them in a higher position, indicating respect. The position of the uncle indicates a more distant relative with some sense of recognition of his role as an older member of the family. Typically, older family members are placed above the client when the roles in the family follow traditional Western cultural pathways in family history. The husband's most distant relationship is with his paternal grandparents. The closest relationships for the husband are with his parents and pet.

There is some slight distance between both partners from the emotional center. The child seems prominently placed with a relatively large symbol size in the center of the family symbol. We do see some color clustering in this drawing with the wife placing her symbols on the right and the husband mostly on the left. This is not too unusual in couple's drawings. However, in this drawing we do see some evidence of distance between the partners. We can use the placements in the drawing as a way to investigate the meaning of the placements. Regardless of the symbol placements, it is always a good idea to ask the person placing the symbol if the therapist's or facilitator's guesses about relationship connections and cutoffs are accurate assumptions.

STEP FIVE: ENVIRONMENTAL SYMBOLS

Key to Symbols (Husband)

Work: side job he enjoys
W: work for income
Fl: family life
WA: spending time at water

MB: mountain biking
YW: yard work
F: faith

Key to Symbols (Wife)

C: church
H: house
Hob: hobbies

HW: husband's jobs and work

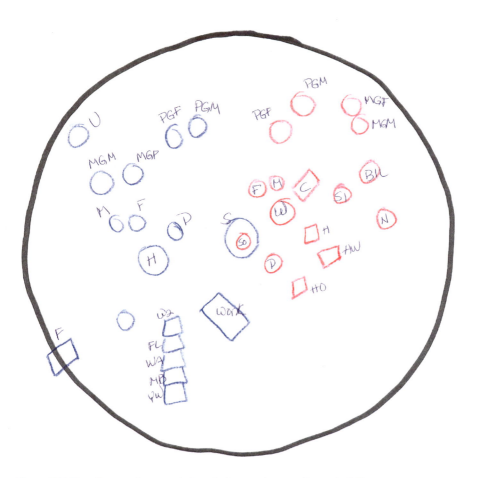

Figure 7.7 Step five, environmental symbols: couple case, Example 7.B

Table 7.8 Step five, environmental symbols: zones, regions, size, and distance, Example 7.B

Husband	Wife
Outside: partial symbol for faith 8:00	Outside: no symbols
Outer: partial faith 8:00, yard work 7:00, partial MB 7:00	Outer: no symbols
Middle: Work 6:00, family life 7:00, water activities 7:00, partial MT biking 7:00	Middle: partial C 3:00
Inner: W 6:00	Inner: house 3:00–4:00, husband's work 3:00–4:00, hobbies 4:00
Size: symbols are smaller with the exception of large work and large faith symbol	Size: symbols are similar to her size or smaller

Placement

The husband places his environmental factors mostly in the middle zone of the family symbol. The symbol for his work related to steady income is placed mostly in the inner zone with a small corner of the symbol in the middle zone. The placement is located below his own symbol and is located close to the 6:00 region of the control circle. Other symbols for his work and hobbies are also located in the lower half of the circle in the middle zone close to the 7:00 region of the control circle. The symbol for yard work is located in the upper edge of the outer zone. One symbol is located in the outer zone and that is the symbol for his faith. The symbol is half in and half out of the family symbol. That symbol is located in the 8:00 position of the control circle. He states that he was raised in a Christian church but considers himself to currently be an agnostic. The environmental symbols are not remarkable in and of themselves, but they are larger than the symbols he placed for people. His symbol for his steady job and his symbol for faith are the largest symbols in his drawing.

The wife places her symbols close to the inner circle with house located directly below her symbol inside the inner circle. The symbol for her husband's work is located in the inner zone near the 4:00 position. Her symbol for hobbies intersects the inner circle and the middle zone. She comments that she does not have so much time for hobbies such as reading and exercising since the birth of the baby. These symbols are close to the 3:00 and 4:00 region of the control circle. Her symbol for church is located slightly above her symbol to the right and places this symbol intersecting the edge of the inner circle and the middle zone. Just above the 3:00 position She indicates that she was raised in the Christian faith but has not practiced actively with a community, but that it is still "close" to her.

Distance

Most of the husband's environmental symbols are located relatively close to the symbol that the husband draws for himself. He locates his steady job as 2.5 cm from his symbol and his second job, which he enjoys more, at 3 cm from his symbol. Below the symbol for his enjoyable second job, he places symbols for family life at 3.2 cm and a symbol for his hobby of being near the water at 3.8 cm and his symbol for mountain biking at 4.5 cm followed by the symbol for yard work at 5 cm. The symbol for faith while located in and out of the family symbol is 4 cm away from his own symbol.

Table 7.9 Step five: distances, husband, Example 7.B

Work	Work2	Family life	Water activities	MT biking	Yard work	Faith
2.5 cm	3 cm	3.2	3.8 cm	4.5 cm	5 cm	4 cm

Table 7.10 Step five: distances, wife, Example 7.B

Church 1.3 cm	House 1.2 cm	Hobbies 2.7 cm	Husband's work 2.3 cm

Reflections on Step Five: Couples Case Example 7.B

The husband has a lot of activities to manage along with the adjustments of a new family. Looking at these environmental symbols, we can begin to see that adjustments in lifestyle after the birth of the new baby might be a factor in the current situation between himself and his wife. Investigating his experiences with these symbols helps to clarify counseling needs.

The wife places her symbols close to the emotional center and close to her. She would place emotional significance to these activities and would be most likely affected by the issues connected to them.

The baby is placed in the emotional center by both of the new parents. Unfortunately, the symbol for the baby appears to be between their symbols possibly representing their marital discord. Investigating these symbolic placements can open up discussion about adjustments for the couple after the baby's birth.

STEP SIX: STRESS SYMBOLS

After placing symbols for environmental factors in the family life space, the facilitator or therapist demonstrates the symbol for stress and invites the partners to place symbols for stress that affects the family. The couple is reminded that stress is often considered negative but stress can also be pressure about positive features in life.

This couple placed symbols related to their relationship and with issues related to the husband's work and hobbies.

Key to Symbols

Husband   **Wife**

R: relationship   R: Relationship
C: commuting
W: wife

Reflections on Step Six (Husband): Couple Case Example 7.B
Placement

The husband placed the stress symbols for all of his symbols in the inner circle of the family drawing. This is a possible indication of the emotional significance of the stresses. He places a symbol for the relationship stress with his wife just above his symbol for his son in the 12:00 zone of the control circle. This is an indication that the stress is significant to his emotional sense of well-being. He places another symbol near the lower edge of the inner zone just above his work symbol and indicates that it is for commuting in traffic to his place of employment. That symbol is located between the 7:00 zone of the control circle. He has a stress symbol for his wife just over the symbol that the wife placed for herself. He indicates that he is concerned because she does not seem happy with him and he is concerned for her stress.

Size

These symbols are average in size, but what is most notable is that the largest stress symbol in the drawing is connected to his wife.

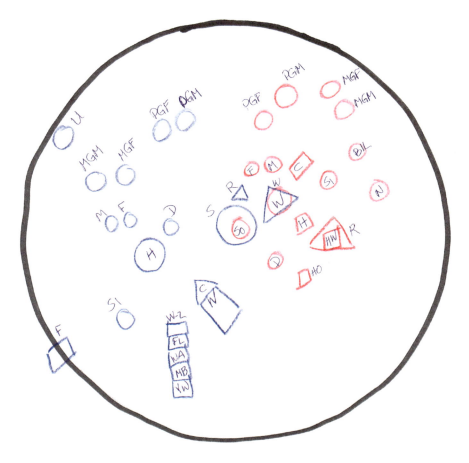

Figure 7.8 Step six, stress symbols: couple case, Example 7.B

Table 7.11 Step six, stress symbols: zone, region, size, and distance, Example 7.B

Husband	Wife
Zone and region Relationship: inner 12:00 Commuting: inner 7:00 Wife: inner 3:00 **Size:** large symbol for wife stress **Distance** wife 4.5 cm, 3.3 cm, commuting 1.5 cm	**Zone and region** Relationship: inner 3:00 **Size:** Similar to other symbols **Distance** relationship 1.6 cm

Distance

The farthest stress symbol for the husband is the stress symbol for his wife, located at 4.5 cm from his symbol. The closest symbol is the symbol for commuting stress. We see that these symbols are located near the symbols for the issues of concern and most likely relate to the rationale behind the placement of the symbol.

Reflections on Step Six (Wife): Couple Case Example 7.B
Placement

The one symbol placed by the wife is located in the inner circle of the control zone slightly below the 3:00 region of the circle. One corner of the symbol is located in the middle zone. She places a stress symbol over the symbol for her husband's jobs and work.

Size

The symbol for stress is larger in size to other symbols she placed in this drawing, other than the symbol placed for self.

Distance

The symbol is located close to her own symbol but below her symbol for self.

Reflections

What stands out in this drawing is the lack of symbols for other stressors. The wife expressed her concern about the husband's activities and did not add other stressors. It would be good to attempt a questioning line that would ask about other stressors, such as adjusting to change of life related to being a new mother and leaving her profession to be a stay-at-home mother and stresses in the marital relationship.

STEP SEVEN: NUMBER ONE CONCERN AND GREATEST FRUSTRATION (NOT ILLUSTRATED)

Husband's number one concern is that they have a happy relationship and his worries about the problems they are currently having. The wife echoes this concern in placing her symbol for number one concern near the husband's similar symbol. Both place these symbols in the inner circle near the center in the 12:00 region of the control circle.

The greatest frustration for him is managing his life's interests. He wants to provide a steady income but is interested in pursuing the farm work. She placed a symbol on top of his, saying that she is frustrated that he is not sure of what he wants to do. He placed this symbol just below his symbol located in the inner zone. The wife's greatest frustration is the uncertainty of the future and wondering how they will manage the new child and work for both of them. This symbol is placed in the lower section of the inner circle near the 6:00 zone.

USING THIS DRAWING WITH THIS COUPLE CASE EXAMPLE 7.B

The FLSD process has an opportunity to explore the meaning of the symbols with the couple by asking more questions about the symbols in the drawing. It would be important to understand the pattern of interaction the couple has developed around these difficult topics. The drawing shows us a distance between the couple with both locating on opposite sides of the inner zone possibly reflecting conflict and disconnections in the relationship. Guiding the couple toward improved connection would be a treatment goal. Reflecting on these symbols helps the couple and therapist or counselor to develop a treatment plan by exploring more information about the symbols as it relates to work stress and investigating underlying desires and longings related to their frustrations and concerns.

Couple Case Example 7.C

The next FLSD is an example of an unmarried couple who have a baby together. They have lived together but recently have separated and are seeking counseling to help them make some decisions about their relationship. The couple have been in relationship for 4 years. The female client, a 35-year-old Caucasian American of southern European descent, contacted the therapist to seek relationship counseling with her on-and-off partner. The male partner is a 38-year-old Caucasian American also of southern European descent. The female was not certain if the romantic relationship would proceed, but she knew that the two of them would have to figure out how to parent the daughter that they shared together. Recently, the couple separated after living together for the last 3 years. The separation was due to her recent discovery that he had been conducting an affair with his ex-wife, the mother of his son born about the same time as the couple's daughter.

The female has a living married mother and father who live several hours away from her. The female is the youngest of five siblings who live in various places across the United States. The female is divorced and has one daughter with special needs from that previous marriage. The child has very little contact with her biological father.

The male is also divorced and has one child born from this relationship after his separation from his spouse, who is also the mother of this child. He has living parents who are married to each other and live about three hours away from his home location. He had a connection to his deceased grandparents who were close to him while he was growing up. He describes his family as close-knit. He is the youngest of two siblings and has one older sister who also lives near his parents.

Both describe their relationship as extremely passionate and difficult to resist. They met when they were working in the same facility but no longer work at the same place of employment. He was married when they met and left his wife to pursue a relationship with this woman, identified as the female. Recently he has been seeing more of his ex-wife in relation to parenting visits. He expresses ambivalence about which woman he wishes to be committed to in a relationship. Both women have asked him to make a decision, and he is unable to decide which relationship is more significant to him.

Step Three: Placement of Self

In step three, each member of the couple is asked to come to the board and place symbols to represent where they see themselves in this family they have formed together.

FLSD: EXAMPLES WITH COUPLES | 115

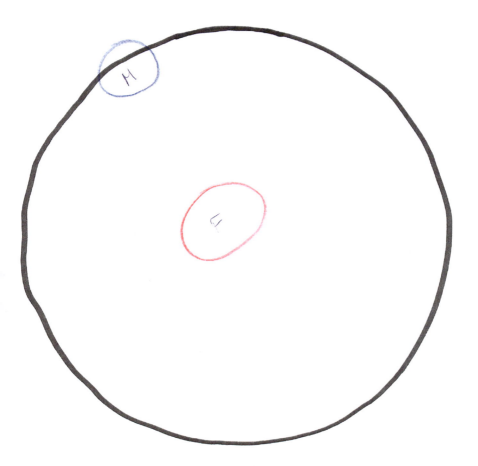

Figure 7.9 Step three, placing individual symbol: couple case, Example 7.C

Key to Symbols

M: male   F: female

Table 7.12 Step three: placement of symbol for self, Example 7.C

Male: blue	Female: red
Placement: Partially located outside the family symbol and mostly located in the outer zone at 11:00	**Placement**: center of the inner zone, covering all regions
Size: symbol size is large enough to cover the 11:00 region	**Size**: symbol is large enough to cover a large part of inner zone

Reflections on Step Three: Couple Case Example 7.C

The female places herself in the center of the inner circle. This indicates a sense of emotional connection and responsibility to the sense she has of family. The male in this couple placed himself in the upper left-hand side of the family symbol. He is located in the 11:00 position with a very large part of him located mostly in the outer zone of the control circle. Part of his symbol is located outside the family symbol.

STEP FOUR: PLACEMENT OF SIGNIFICANT OTHERS

After the second person in the couple has placed a symbol to represent their place in the family, the person is asked to place symbols for other people significant to the family. In this situation, the couple have children and parents to represent. The female has a 5-year-old daughter from a previous relationship, who has special needs and requires extra services in school and specialized medical care. In addition to her daughter from her marriage, she is caring for their baby living with her in the home previously shared with the male. There are other family members in this family represented in the key below.

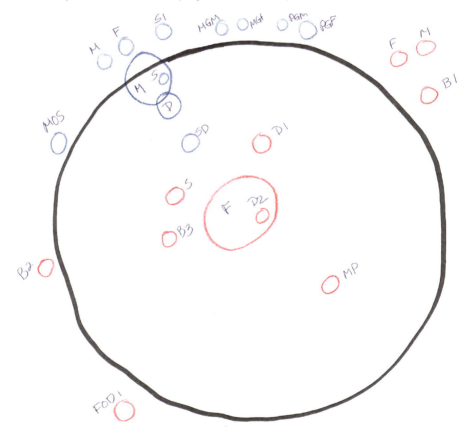

Figure 7.10 Step four, placing significant others: couple case, Example 7.C

Key to Symbols

Female

D1: daughter 1, age 5
D2: 18-month-old
Sister
Brother 3
Brother 2

M: mother
F: father
B1: brother 1
FD: father of daughter
MP: male partner

Male

S: son, 18 months old
D: daughter
SD: stepdaughter
MOS: mother of son
MGF: maternal grandfather
PGM: paternal grandmother

M: mother
F: father
S: sister
MGM: Maternal grandmother
PGF: Paternal grandfather

Table 7.13 Step four, significant others: zone, region, size, and distance, Example 7.C

Female: red	Male: blue
Outside Father 1:00, Brother1 2:00, Brother2 9:00 Mother 1:00, Father of Daughter 7:00	Outside Mother of Son 10:00, MGM 12:00 Mother 11:00, MGF 12:00 Father 11:00, PGM 12:00 Sister 11:00, PGF 12:00
Outer No symbols	Outer Son, inside his symbol at 11:00 Daughter, partial inside his symbol and partial outer 11:00
Middle: some partial placements Male partner 4:00, Sister 9:00 Brother3 8:00, Daughter1 12:00	Middle: Daughter: partial 11:00 Stepdaughter: 11:00
Inner partial placement Male partner 4:00, Sister 9:00 Brother3 9:00, Daughter1 12:00 Daughter2, inside her symbol 1:00	Inner No symbols
Size: symbols are smaller than her own symbol; children small	Size: symbols for others smaller than his own
Distance Male Partner 2 cm, Brother1 8.2 cm, Daughter1 0.5 cm Brother3 0.1 cm Father 7.8 cm, Brother2 6.3 cm, Daughter2 0 cm Mother 9.5 cm Father of daughter 8.3 cm Sister1 0.2 cm	Distance Son 0 cm, Sister 2 cm PGM 5 cm Mother 2.2 cm, MGM 3.8 cm Daughter 0 cm, Father 2 cm PGM 5.1 cm Stepdaughter 1.5 cm MGF 4 cm, PGF 6.4 cm Mother of daughter 3 cm

Reflections on Step Four (Female Placements): Couple Case Example 7.C

The female's youngest daughter is placed inside in the upper right-hand side and edge the female's symbol, possibly indicating a lack of differentiation or possible emotional issues connected to this child. The female's older daughter is located just above the female's symbol for self toward the 12:00 zone of the control circle. Other symbols located in the inner circle are symbols for her brother who is located to the left of her symbol just below the 9:00 position. Also, partially in the inner zone is a symbol for the sister, who is located above and to the left of the symbol for the female toward the 11:00 zone of the control circle.

The middle zone of this drawing contains a symbol for the male partner, who is located partially in the inner zone as well. He is located in the 4:00 zone of the control circle. The female does not place any symbols in the outer zone but does place some symbols outside of the family symbol.

Several family members are located outside of the family symbol. These include some significant family members such as mother and father and some siblings. The father and mother are located outside of the family symbol in the upper right-hand section of the drawing near the 1:00 position. Her oldest brother is also located near them below the parents closer to the 2:00 position. On the other side of the drawing located outside the family symbol near the 9:00 position is a symbol for her second oldest brother. In the lower half of the drawing outside the family symbol the female has drawn her ex-husband, the father of her oldest daughter.

The size of the symbol that the female draws for herself is a relatively large symbol when compared to her other symbols. Her symbol almost takes up all of the space in the inner circle. This could be indicative of a large personality or a strong sense of self. Symbols for all the others are close in size to each other with the exception of the two daughters who are smaller in size.

The female's drawing shows some symbols of people extremely close to her symbol and symbols of people very distant. The children in the inner circle have either no distance or minimal distance, with Daughter 1 located 0.5 cm away from the female's symbol for self. The other symbols in the inner circle are 0.4 cm for the sister and similar distance for Brother3.

The male partner has 2 cm of distance in this section, making him the farthest symbol inside the family symbol for the female. Outside the family symbol are the mother at 9.5 cm away and the father at 7.8 cm away. The father of Daughter 1 is far away from the female's symbol in the drawing, placing him at 7.5 cm away from her symbol of self.

It appears that the female has some disconnections in her family of origin. She places her parents above her but outside of her family. She reports that her parents are unhappy with her due to the relationship she has with the male and having a child without being married. She also indicates that some of her siblings have been unsupportive, such as Brother1, and that Brother 2 has his own problems. Even though she is experiencing some frustration with the male, she places him inside the family circle even if it is in a lower place. Please note that we normally do not have people include partners or relatives who are in the room at the time of the drawing. Sometimes clients will spontaneously draw symbols for family members in the room as in this situation. She has a strong sense of self and some supportive connections with some family members, and this element is seen as a strength.

Reflections on Step Four (Male Placements): Couple Case Example 7.C

The male places his son inside his own symbol and places his daughter at the bottom of his symbol intersecting inside his symbol but also outside in in the outer and middle zone. The daughter's symbol is located closer to the 10:00 position. The rest of the male's symbols are located outside the family symbol. He places his ex-wife and mother of his son outside the 10:00 position. He places his parents next to each other above his 11:00 position and slightly to the left. His sister is just above his position and his parents position. Out of the family symbol but above the 12:00 position the male places both sets of grandparents. They are located in a high position but not in this family symbol.

The size of the largest symbol drawn by the male is the symbol for himself. The next largest symbol is for his sister. The symbol for the mother of his son would be next in size. The symbols for his parents and grandparents are similar in size. The symbols for the children are the smallest symbols he draws for people.

The symbols drawn by the male are located close to his own symbol. He draws his children without any distance and his son as a part of him entirely. His mother is 1 cm and his father is 1 cm. The sister is also 2 cm, following a similar pattern to his parents. The mother of his son is placed at 2.5 cm from his own symbol. The grandparents are farthest away. Both sets of grandparents are deceased but he indicates that he was close to both sets. He indicates that he knew his maternal grandparents better than the paternal ones. He is 3 cm away from his maternal grandparents and about 5 cm from his paternal grandmother and 6 cm from his paternal grandfather.

The male's ambivalence toward making a family with the female is visually seen in this drawing by his position of in and out of the family symbol. He does not place his family of origin in the family symbol and keeps them close to him near the outside of the family symbol.

He is close to his family of origin but is keeping these family members away from his connection to the female. He positions himself in a distant but powerful position. The male drawing shows lack of differentiation with his concepts of the children and no separation between him and his 2-year-old son.

STEP FIVE: ENVIRONMENTAL SYMBOLS

After all the symbols for significant others have been placed on this drawing, the facilitator or therapist explains "we will add environmental symbols of things that affect the family but do not necessarily include people. These symbols usually include things like employment, hobbies, organizations, and spiritual practice." This couple each placed symbols for environmental factors that affect their daily life This couple placed symbols for their spiritual practice and symbols for work and hobbies.

USING FLSD WITH DIFFERENT TYPES OF CLIENTS

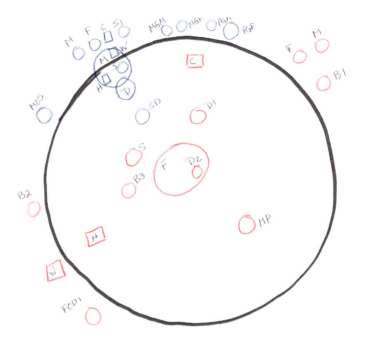

Figure 7.11 Step five, environmental symbols: couple case, Example 7.C

Key to Symbols

Female's   Male

C: church   W: work
H: hobbies   H: hobbies
W: work   C: church

Table 7.14 Step five, environmental symbols: zone, region, size, and distance, Example 7.C

Female	Male
Outside:	Outside:
work 8:00	work 11:00, church 11:00
Outer:	Outer:
church 12:00	hobbies 11:00
hobbies partial 8:00	
Middle:	Middle:
Hobbies partial 8:00	No symbols
Inner:	Inner:
No symbols	No symbols
Size: similar in size smaller than her own symbol	Size: symbols are smaller than his own symbol
Distance:	Distance:
Work 7.2 cm, hobbies 3.2 cm, church 4 cm	work 0 cm, hobbies 0 cm, church 0.5 cm

Reflections on Step Five (Female): Couple Case Example 7.C

The female in this couple has not placed any environmental symbols in the inner zone. One symbol for hobbies straddles the middle and outer zone in the 8:00 region of the control circle. In the upper 12:00 region of the outer zone is a symbol for church that touches the middle zone. These symbols are relatively the same size and do not indicate any remarkable feature to their size. Her hobbies are located in a negative position at 3 cm from her symbol, and church is located about 4 cm from her symbol. Work is located the farthest away at 7.2 cm and in a negative position outside the family symbol.

Even though the symbol for church is in the outer zone, it is located in the 12:00 position, indicating that it is important or significant to her. The placement of work outside the lower part of the circle indicates that it is not held in high regard by the female. She originally met her boyfriend at work and she ended up changing jobs due to the scandals at work. She does not currently have positive feelings about the current work placement.

Reflections on Step Five (Male): Couple Case Example 7.C

The male followed his placements for people by placing his environmental symbols close to the symbol he drew for himself. His symbols for work and hobbies are located inside the symbol that he drew for himself. The symbol for church is located directly above his symbol.

The symbols for hobbies and work are very small. The symbol for church is comparable to his symbols for his parents. The smaller size usually indicates that the institution is not a significant place in his life.

The environmental symbols are very close his own symbol with two of the symbols showing no separation. One symbol for work is at the top of his symbol and the symbol for hobbies is at the bottom of his symbol. The symbol for church is 0.5 cm away from his symbol. The placement and size of the symbols for work and hobbies might indicate that these elements of his life are an integral part of him. He possibly sees no difference between himself and these activities. The combination of all of these placements show a possible emotional intensity connected to his activities.

STEP SIX: STRESS SYMBOLS

After each partner has placed symbols for environmental factors that are a part of the family, the therapist or facilitator draws a triangle and informs that this symbol represents the issues of stress that affect the family. After demonstrating the symbol on a separate piece of paper, the therapist/facilitator will ask each partner to place symbols for stress where each sees it affecting the family. The couple is reminded that stress symbols do not always have to represent negative issues but can represent issues that are important and of concern to the person.

This couple decided to let this drawing reflect the point of their concern. They were coming to the session to work through a relationship crisis and indicated symbols that reflected that concern. They both placed just a few symbols that reflected the stress of the moment. At this point in the process the couple was more relaxed about sharing the history of their current situation. They had been connecting with the therapist through the process of sharing family history and current activities affecting their lives. At this point in the process, it was easier to talk about the presenting issues that drew them to seek counseling in the first place. The drawing process of interacting with the therapist set the stage for comfortable sharing about the difficult topic of the relationship, family relations and the affair.

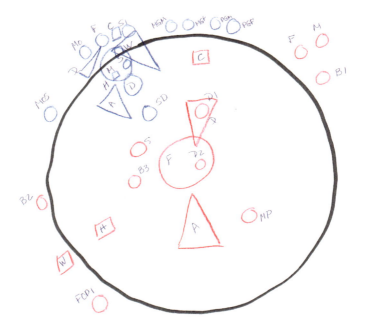

Figure 7.12 Step six, stress symbols: couple case, Example 7.C

Key to Symbols

Female

A: affair
D1: concerns about special needs of daughter 1

Male

W: work
D: stress with dad
A: affair

Reflections on Step Six (Female): Couple Case Example 7.C

The female places her symbols for stress close to her in the inner circle. The tips of the stress symbol point to the symbol she has drawn for herself. The symbols also cross over into the space of the middle and inner zone. The symbols for her concerns for her daughter are located in the 12:00 region of the control zone. On the opposite side of the symbol for herself holds the symbol for the affair at the 6:00 region of the control circle. Both of these stress symbols take on the image of arrows pointing at her.

The symbol size for both stressors is relatively large taking up a lot of space in the family symbol. Once again, the distance between these symbols and the female's symbol is very close. The symbol for the daughter's concern intersects with her own symbol and is located

Table 7.15 Step six, stress symbols: zone, region, size, and distance, Example 7.C

Female	Male
Outside: No symbols	Outside: Father stress 10:00 Work 11:00 partial
Outer: No symbols	Outer: Work 11:00 partial Affair 10:00 partial
Middle: Daughter1 12:00 partial placement Affair 6:00 partial placement	Middle: Work 11:00 partial point Affair 10:00 partial
Inner: Daughter1 12:00 partial placement Affair 6:00 partial placement	Inner: No symbols
Size: large symbols	Size: these are large symbols comparable to his own
Distance: The symbols are close to her with no distance The furthest point of Affair 3.5 cm Daughter 13 cm	Distance: Father stress 1 cm Affair 0 cm distance to 2.7 cm

above her indicating its significance. The symbol for the affair does not touch her but is located in a negative position about 0.2 cm away from her own symbol, reflecting her deep emotional experience and dissatisfaction with it.

These symbols indicate significant stress in her life as illustrated by their placement in the inner circle and the position of 12:00 for her concerns for her daughter showing a significantly more important stress location. The stress around the affair also shows significant placement but slightly less than her concerns for her daughter.

Reflections on Step Six (Male): Couple Case Example 7.C

The only stress that intersects with his symbol for self is the symbol for work. This symbol is placed inside his symbol in the upper right-hand corner. His other stress symbols are close to him. The symbol for the affair is located in the outer zone crossing into the middle zone of the family symbol, near the 10:00 region. This stress symbol is located below the symbol he drew for himself. The only other symbol is his drawing is the symbol for stress with his father. This symbol is located outside the family symbol near the 11:00 position of the male's symbol. The symbol points to the symbol that he drew for his father.

The symbol sizes are large when compared to the other symbols he has created in this FLSD. The largest stress symbol is for work. The work stress symbol is larger than the symbol he drew for work itself. The stress symbol for work also takes in the work symbol. The large stress around work is most likely related to the changes he had to make at work after having his affair with his co-worker, now the female in the session. The workplace affair created problems with his superiors, who have been hesitant to give him more responsibility.

The male's stress symbols are also close to the symbol he drew for himself. Work intersects with his own symbol. The stress symbol for the affair is 0.2 cm away and the symbol for stress with his dad is 0.3 cm away from his own symbol. These stressors are significant for this male client and equal the intensity of all his placements. He places the stress symbol with the affair in the family symbol and it is the closest symbol to his partner's symbol. His drawing does indicate that he is keeping this family separate from his family of origin and other family. He did indicate that his parents were very unhappy that he had left his wife to have a relationship with the female in this drawing and that his stress with his father is related to that life event. There is some concern illustrated in this drawing that the male partner may not be able to make a strong investment to the family with this female in this drawing.

Using the FLSD With Couple Case Example 7.C

While in the process of completing this drawing, the couple was able to observe that the male partner was on both the outside and inside of the family symbol. The female partner noted that and expressed concern about his commitment to her. The couple and therapist recognized that treatment would focus on the issue of making a decision about the commitment to the relationship. The symbolic representations allowed the clients to express concerns about the effects on other family members and helped to define the serious issues concerning this family. The emotional cutoffs with the female's family of origin were noted and observed as making it difficult for her to have family support that she needs, especially with a special needs child. The drawing was an excellent launching pad in beginning the identification of clarifying treatment issues and beginning the process of making decisions about the future of their relationship. It was clear that the female was not ready to let go of this relationship and that time and counseling needed to help her define relationship boundaries and expectations. Both members of the couple illustrated this drawing with emotional intensity and reflected that the people, places, and issues related to their lives were very close and experienced with a sense of importance. Focusing on the positive nature of the intensity and the visual representations will help this couple develop a treatment path.

Summary of Using FLSD With Couples

The FLSD can be utilized with almost any type of family arrangement and has the benefit of adapting to all family forms. The use of the FLSD with couples help the partners to see how the individual issues intersect with each other in helping to clarify the issues that brought the couple into therapy in the first place. This chapter illustrated the use of the FLSD as a first session tool helping couples to share introductory information while connecting with the therapist in the therapeutic process. The process helps to avoid common issues in couple's therapy where individuals will take up more time in the session to share their story. The FLSD is more likely to facilitate equal time for sharing information and direct contact with the therapist to facilitate an equal sense of alliance with each member of the couple.

CHAPTER EIGHT
Family Life Space Drawing With Families

FAMILIES AND THE FLSD

Using the FLSD is an ideal way to meet families engaging in counseling for the first time. The FLSD is a process whereby each family member contributes to the intake information obtained by the therapist. The process works by providing individual, direct attention to all of the people in the family. After each family member has an individual opportunity to present family information, all of the individual information combines in the final picture of the FLSD. At the completion point of the FLSD, the individuals in the family have created a bird's-eye view of their family system and we see the individual parts combined in an artful mosaic that gives everyone a sense of the whole family situation. It is much like viewing the planet earth from the spaceship. We see the whole picture of the sometimes-fragile space that holds all the family members and their struggles that bring them to therapy.

Conducting the FLSD with a large family group can take a long time, and it is important to set aside enough time to let the process evolve. The process can take up to two hours to complete but can be completed in the limits of normal therapy sessions. It is important to ask questions and to provide each person in the family group an opportunity to obtain enough attention to allow for the sense of connection and engagement with the therapist that is so crucial to the family therapy process.

The final drawing of a family group can often look like an example of modern art with shapes, colors, and lines. This often messy visual needs a careful step-by-step processing to see how the drawing proceeds with each individual placement and the final conclusion of the whole family picture. People in families often enjoy applying their symbols; even family members who did not think they would speak in the session often end up as active participants in the process and looking on with excited interest as others draw their symbols.

In this chapter, we provide examples of two families seeking family treatment. The first family is a blended family that was interested in helping the children work on adjustments to blending two families. The second example reveals a family that sought treatment for one issue related to a child's behavior but learned in the first session that the problem was broader than they first suspected.

BLENDED FAMILY: CASE EXAMPLE 8.A

This example illustrates a combined family drawing of six family members who are in the early process of forming a family group. The man and the woman each have two children and after dating several years, decided to get married and combine their two families together into the same home. This is a demonstration of a large family group.

The woman has primary custody of her children, a son age 10 and a daughter age 8. The female in this family jointly divides parenting time with the children's father who lives nearby. She was married to her children's father, who is a native-born American of northern European descent. The woman and the children's father have been able to work harmoniously as they co-parent their children. The woman's parents live nearby and are able to help her with after school childcare for the children. The woman has a profession in high-tech and immigrated to this country from eastern Europe to work in that profession. Her parents were able to join her in the United States and she has lived here for 12 years.

The new husband in this drawing has two sons aged 10 and 6 and is an immigrant from India who also works in the high-tech profession. He has lived in the United States for 12 years. He was previously married to an American woman of northern European descent and she is the mother of his children. The new husband has his parents living nearby and his parents interact with this family group on a regular basis. The children have some grandparents on their mother's side but they do not interact very often as the grandparents live far away.

The recently married couple sought out counseling to help the children work on adjustments to the new family configuration. The man's ex-wife was having some difficulty concerning the recent marriage and was causing some distress in the family. The new couple wanted to help the children with the adjustment of now living together even though the children knew each other well and interacted on weekends and family vacations for several years. The parents were confident of the children's friendship but wanted the new changes in living space to go as smoothly as possible.

Step Three: Placement of Self

Key to Symbols

F: female lt blue
M: male dk blue
MS1: male's son 1 green
MS2: male's son 2 orange
FS: female's son brown
FD: female's daughter purple

In step three, each family member places themselves individually in the life space drawing. In this instance, the family drawing includes: The adults identified as male and female and the children identified as male son 1 and male son 2 and female's son and female's daughter.

Reflections on Step Three: Family Case Example 8.A

The most striking observation about the placements of family members in this drawing is noticing the absence of anyone in the emotional center of the family drawing. Typically, we will see at least one parent place themselves in the family center but in this situation, we see no one. Seeing this image, suggests that the family is still in the process of forming a family unit of identity. Parents are still in the process of incorporating their expanded roles as not only parents but now stepparents. The other notable observation in this drawing has to do with the placement of male son 1. He is located in a location that is somewhat isolated from other family members in a high large symbol that is different from other family symbols. When children draw larger symbols for themselves it can mean that

FAMILY LIFE SPACE DRAWING WITH FAMILIES | 127

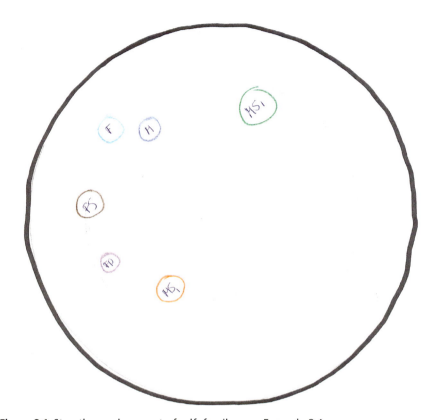

Figure 8.1 Step three, placement of self: family case, Example 8.A

Table 8.1 Step three, placement of self: zone, region, and size, Example 8.A

	Male: dark blue	Female: light blue	Male's son 1: green	Male's son 2: orange	Female's son: brown	Female's daughter: purple
placement	Middle zone 10:00	Outer zone border on middle 10:00	Middle zone 12:00	Middle zone inner zone between 6:00–7:00	Middle zone touching outer 9:00	Middle zone 8:00
Size	Average size	Average size	large	Average	Average	Average

they have a parental child position or that they feel a sense of power or responsibility in the family. Most of the time this power is not appropriate and can create stress for the child. This child has been verbally identified by the parents and the other children as a positive and negative attention seeker. This child often tends to be a family leader. In this FLSD session he was often drawing attention to himself by making noises and comments even when it was not his turn to be at the drawing board. The structured process of the FLSD can be helpful when working with attention seeking family members because it allows the therapist facilitator to remind the participants that they will have a turn soon. When the attention seeker has their turn at the board, special attention can be given to that person in a positive way.

Step Four: Placement of Significant Others

After each family member has had an opportunity to place their own individual symbol, the last person up at the board is asked to add other people who are in the family but not currently in the room. In this family children would be asked to place the parent or relatives who are not in the room as well as any other significant people.

Key to Symbols

Male: dk blue

MM: male's mother
MF: male's father
S: sister
P: pet
CM: children's mother

Female: lt blue

FM: female's mother
FF: female's father
B: brother MS: sister in-law
Pet
CF: children's father
M: husband's mother
MF: husband's father

Green: male son 1

M: mother
PGM: paternal grandfather
PGF: paternal grandmother
MGM: maternal grandmother
Maternal grandfather
Female's mother
Female's father
A: aunt
P: pet
Brown: female's son
Dad: father
MGM: maternal grandmother
MGF: maternal grandfather
PGM: paternal grandfather
PGF: paternal grandmother
MlM: males mother
MLF: males father
P: pet

Orange: male son 2

M: mother
MGM: maternal grandmother
MGF: maternal grandfather
PGM: paternal grandmother
PGF: paternal grandfather
Female's mother
Female's father
Aunt
P: pet
Purple: female's daughter
Dad: father
MGM: maternal grandmother
MGF: maternal grandfather
PGM: paternal grandmother
PGF: maternal grandfather
MLM: male's mother
MLF: male's father
P: pet

Reflections on Step Four: Family Case Example 8.A

Adding significant others to this drawing is a time to gather information about other family members not present in the room. The drawing allows for the children to report nonverbally about their parents. The male's children visually demonstrate that their mother is a large

FAMILY LIFE SPACE DRAWING WITH FAMILIES | 129

Table 8.2 Step four, significant others: zone placements, Example 8.A

Male: dark blue	Female: light blue	MS1: green	MS2: orange	FS: orange	FD: purple
Outside: No symbols	Outside: No symbols	Outside: No symbols	Outside: No symbols	Outside: No symbols	Outside: No symbols
Outer: Mother 12:00 Father 12:00 Children's mother between 4:00–5:00	Outer: Mother 11:00 Father 11:00 Male's mother 12:00 Male's father 12:00 Brother 9:00 Children's father between 7:00–8:00	Outer: PGM right of 12:00 PGF right of 12:00 MGM 2:00 MGF 2:00 Female's mother 10:00 Female's Father 10:00	Outer: Female's mother 9:00 Female's Father 9:00	Outer: PGM 9:00 PGF 9:00	Outer: Dad 8:00 MGM 8:00, partially in middle zone MGF 8:00 PGM 8:00 PGF 8:00
Middle: No symbols	Middle: Male's sister 10:00	Middle: Mom taking some of the space of the outer and inner zone	Middle: MGF 6:00 MGF 6:00	Middle: MGM 9:00 MGF 9:00 Dad 9:00 Male's mother and male's father Slightly lower 9:00	Middle: Pet 8:00
Inner: Pet close to 5:00	Inner: Pet 6:00	Inner: Aunt 10:00 Pet 12:00–1:00	Inner: Mom 8:00 Pet 6:00 Aunt 12:00 PGM 12:00 PGF 12:00	Inner: Pet is on edge of inner at 9:00	Inner: no symbols

presence in the family. Son1 has his mother in a powerful position and also has her taking up some space in the inner, middle, and outer zone. Son2 sees the mother in a lower position but still large in the family center. She is positioned as the closest symbol to him and occupies a prominent position in the inner zone. Male son1 also has his mother as the closet symbol to him in this drawing. The oldest son places the symbol for his mother on the other side of the family group. The therapist needs to be sensitive to the role that the male's children's mother plays in the family and encourage her potential participation in future family sessions.

The female's son draws his father close to him and locates him close to the inner zone. The daughter sees her Dad in the outer zone. Even with this placement she places him close to her symbol. The therapist would also be wise to investigate the father of the female's children role in the new emerging family.

In the course of completing this drawing we discover that the female and her children used to live with the maternal grandparents. The grandparents still provide babysitting and back up care to the children and are an active part of the children's lives. Both children locate their grandparents close to them and above them showing respect. The Female's son sees them in an upper position and places them highest of all his symbols.

The male's children place grandparents more distantly. The paternal grandparents for male Son 2 are the farthest away. Even though he does see them distantly from his own symbol

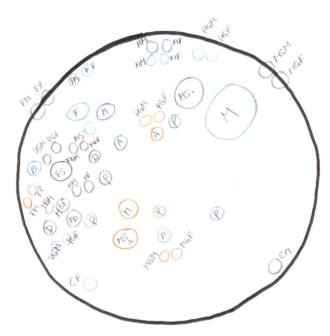

Figure 8.2 Step four, drawing significant others: family case, Example 8.A

Table 8.3 Step four, significant other: size and distance, Example 8.A

Male: dark blue	Female: light blue	MS1: green	MS2: orange	FS: brown	Female daughter: purple
Size: symbols similar in size	Size: smaller than symbol for self, smallest for parents	Size: most symbols smaller than his own symbol Mother's symbol is larger than his	Size: has a large symbol for Mom; the rest are smaller than his symbol	Size: all symbols are smaller than his own symbol	Size: All symbols similar size
Distance: Mother 2.5 cm Father 2.5 cm Sister 1 cm Children's mother 13 cm Pet 8.3 cm	Distance: Mother 1.5 cm Father 2 cm Brother 2.5 cm Male's mother 3.2 cm Male's father 4.2 cm Children's father 8.5 cm Pet 6 cm	Distance: Mom 0.5 cm PGM 1.5 cm PGF 1.5 cm MGM 4 cm MGF 4.5 cm Female's mother 7 cm Female's father 6.5 cm Aunt 3.5 cm	Distance: Mom 0.5 cm Pet 1.4 cm MGM 2 cm MGF 2 cm PGM 6.5 cm PGF 7 cm Aunt 5.5 cm Females mother 6 cm Females father 6.5 cm	Distance: Dad 0.5 cm MGM 1 cm MGF 1.4 cm PGF 0.7 cm PGM 0.6 cm Males mother 0.5 Males father 0.8 Pet 1.5	Distance: Dad 1.5 cm Pet 0.2 MGM 0.7 MGF 0.3 PGM 1.5 PGF 0.6

he places the grandparents in a high position in the inner zone. The oldest male son places grandparents in a higher position above him. They are the only symbols above him and such placements can be indicating respect. While completing the drawing the children share that their maternal grandparents live some distance away and that they do not know them very well. This is illustrated by the oldest son placing his maternal grandparents in a high position of respect but half in and out of the family circle.

Both the adult male and the adult female place their parents above them in the outer zone of the family. This position show respect.

The males' children do have symbols for the Female's parents and they are just getting to know each other. The female's son sees these step grandparents as close to him but underneath his symbol. The oldest son of the male places his step grandparents as his most distantly placed symbol indicating that he is not as close to them but places them in a respectful position. We see the female's daughter following a similar pattern placing her step grandparents in a position of regard but at a distance from her.

Pets present a key placement for the four of the family members in the inner zone. Placing pets in the center is a commonly observed phenomena in families. We suggest that pets are a predictable source of connection and emotional comfort for people.

Noticing placement zone and clock positions on the FLSD help to provide suggestions as to unspoken connections and regards as in this drawing where children may not place symbols close to their own symbol but place the symbol in a high position. An example of this is where you can see in the family drawing: the youngest child placed maternal grandparents that he does not know very well as the lowest positioned people in his drawing. He may place them relatively close but with lesser regard.

The final observation at this phase of the drawing is noticing the pattern of family members placing most of the symbols on the left side. It is getting crowded in that part of the symbol. The oldest son of the male is noticeably in his own side of the drawing.

STEP FIVE: ENVIRONMENTAL SYMBOLS

After the last family member has completed the symbols for significant others, the therapist/facilitator will draw the symbol for environmental factors as a small square and ask that person to draw symbols in the drawing for environmental and institutional issues that affect that individual and the family. These can include things like work, school, hobbies, and spiritual practice. Each person took turns placing their symbols on the drawing and had the followings items placed on the drawing.

Key to Symbols

Male: dk blue

w: work
S: children's school
KA: kids' activities
Spiritual practice
Running

Male's son1: Green

MH: mom's house
Sc: school
So: soccer

Female: lt blue

E: exercise
KA: children's activities
S: children's school
Work
Spiritual practice

Male's son2: orange

Sc: school
S: soccer

USING FLSD WITH DIFFERENT TYPES OF CLIENTS

Female's son: brown

DH: dad's house
SC: school
SO: soccer

Female's daughter: purple

Sc: school
SO: soccer

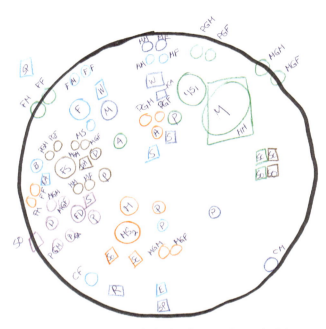

Figure 8.3 Step five, environmental symbols: family case, Example 8.A

Table 8.4 Step five, environmental symbols: placements, regions, and zones, Example 8.A

Male: dark blue	Female: light blue	MS1: green	MS2: orange	FS: brown	FD: purple
Outside: no symbols	Outside: SP 10:00	Outside: no symbols	Outside: no symbols	Outside: no symbols	Outside: Soccer partial 8:00
Outer: R between 6:00 and 7:00 Spiritual practice 6:00	Outer: Kids' activities 9:00 Exercise 6:00	Outer: Partial mom's house 2:00	Outer: no symbols	Outer: School partial out 3:00 Soccer partial 3:00	Outer: Soccer partial 8:00
Middle: work 12:00 Kids' activities 12:00	Middle: no symbols	Middle: Mom's house 2:00 School 3:00 Soccer 3:00	Middle: Soccer 6:00–7:00 School 6:00	Middle: DH 9:00 SC 3:00 SO 3:00	Middle: School 8:00
Inner: S 12:00	Inner: School 12:00	Inner: no symbols	Inner: no symbols	Inner: no symbols	Inner: no symbols

FAMILY LIFE SPACE DRAWING WITH FAMILIES | 133

Table 8.5 Step five, environmental symbols: size and distance, Example 8.A

Male: dark blue	Female: light blue	MS1: green	MS2: orange	FS: brown	FD: purple
Size: symbols smaller than his own symbol	Size: symbols are similar to her own symbol	Size: large symbol for MH Other symbols smaller than his own symbol	Size: symbols smaller than his own symbol. School is largest	Size: symbols are on the small range	Size: symbols are small
Distance: Work 0.5 cm School 2.5 cm Kids' activities 1 cm Spiritual practice 13 cm Running 11 cm	Distance: School 4.8 cm Kids activities 3 cm Work 0.3 cm Exercise 12.3 cm Spiritual practice 4 cm	Distance: School 4.6 cm Soccer 5.7 cm Moms house: 0 cm	Distance: School 0.5 cm Soccer 0.3	Distance: Dad's house 0.2 cm School 11 cm Soccer 12 cm	Distance: School 0.1 cm Soccer 2.2 cm

Reflections on Step Five: Family Case Example 8.A

Overall this family did not place many symbols for environmental elements affecting this family, more often, typical family drawings will include many outside activities and issues affecting the family. This family drawing reveals that family environmental elements are few in number and that they seemed to be managed within the day-to-day activities. Most of the environmental symbols are small and located in outside positions.

The parents of these children placed activities related to the children in the upper half of the family drawing indicating a position of regard and concern. Activities other than work were placed in lower positions in the family drawing. Both adults indicated that their personal activities took a backseat to whatever the children were doing. Both work professionally and experience their work as significant but in a balanced place,

The male and female of this family group indicated that they were both raised as Muslims but they do not have a strong connection to everyday spiritual practice. The female stated that her spiritual belief is important to her personal sense of culture and values but she does not observe a strict observance in her life. None of the children mentioned any influence of spiritual practice in their life.

School seems to be an important issue with the adults in this family as they placed it in the emotional center of the family drawing. Both of the parents are educated and stated that education gave them opportunities. They hope that the children will take advantage of education and continue to do well in school. The placement of the symbols for school near the children indicate a favorable attitude toward education. The two younger children placed school close to their own positions and the two older boys placed school with more distance. The female's oldest son said that he placed school near the symbol of his oldest stepbrother because they would go to same school and be in the same grade. All the children and the parents stated that the children were good students. Male Son 1 did note that sometimes he does not like school because he does not like to sit still and the teachers sometimes get mad at him for making noise in class.

The most notable symbol in this drawing is related to the symbol for Male Son 1's mother's house. The drawing indicates that being at her home is important to this child. This symbol indicates a significant influence for this child and reveals some possible unspoken concerns with being or not being at this house. Through the process of the drawing the child tells us a lot without expressing any words. It is useful to reference this symbol either at this time in the process or after the drawing is completed in order to gain more information as to the symbol's significance. The female "son also drew a symbol for his father's house after seeing Male Son 1 draw his symbol." When noting the difference in the two symbols, The green symbol (male's oldest son) is extra-large and the brown (female's oldest son) symbol is on the small size. We would assume that Dad's house while important to the female's son does not have the significance of the oldest son of the male. The positioning of the mother's house by the male son 1 reinforces the importance of the symbol he placed for his mother. This environmental symbol helps to support the need to be sensitive to the relationship of the male's children's mother with the family.

Once again, this family drawing has most of the family members placing most of the symbols on the left side of the drawing in a crowed cluster almost in an age related semi-circle. Parents are at the top with oldest female son followed by daughter and then the youngest child in this drawing male's youngest son. The oldest son of the male placed his activities off to the right with his stepbrother joining him in activities they share together. This joining could be seen as a positive sign that the female's son does want to connect to his stepbrother through these activities.

Step Six: Stress Symbols

After the last family member has placed the environmental symbols the therapist facilitator draws the triangle symbol representing stress. The therapist facilitator informs the family members that this symbol represents stresses that are affecting the family. In this family, especially with children it is important to reference stress as something that might be a worry or a concern. Family members also need to be reminded that stress is often thought of as a bad thing but it can be something that presses on your mind and is important to you.

Key to Symbols

Male: dk blue

CF: children fighting
M: move
Mo: mother

MS1: green

Mom: concern for Mom
Move

Female's Son brown

SO-Soccer
SC-School
M-Move

Female: lt blue

M: move
Pa: parenting
CS: children's school

MS2: orange

Mom: concern for Mom
School

M-move

Female daughter

S: school
B: boys in house

Reflections on Step Six: Family Case Example 8.A

One of the positive observations in observing this drawing related to stress is that the family seems to have little stress and the stress they have appears to be managed. Most of the stress symbols are relatively smaller than each member's symbol for self. Most of the stress symbols are placed in the lower half of the family drawing possibly indicating that the stress symbols

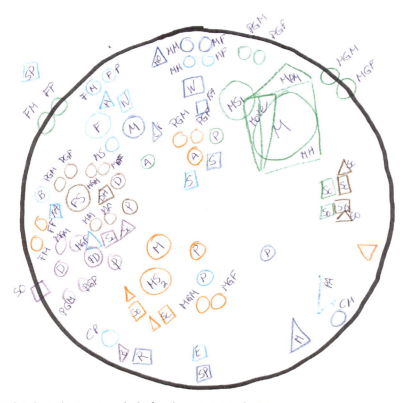

Figure 8.4 Step six, stress symbols: family case, Example 8.A

Table 8.6 Step six: stress symbols, Example 8.A

Male: dark blue	Female: light blue	MS1: green	MS2: orange	FS: brown	FD: purple
Outside: no symbols	Outside: no symbols	Outside: no symbols	Outside: no symbols	Outside: no symbols	Outside: no symbols
Outer: Mother 12:00 Move 5:00–6:00	Outer: Move 10:00 Parenting 5:00	Outer: Mom 1:00	Outer: Move 4:00	Outer: School partial 3:00 Soccer partial 3:00 M 9:00	Outer: Boys 7:00
Middle: Children fighting 11:00	Middle: Partial Parenting 5:00 Children's school 8:00	Middle: Move 12:00–1:00	Middle: Soccer 7:00 School 6:00	Middle: no symbols	Middle: School partial 9:00
Inner: no symbols	Inner:	Inner: no symbols	Inner: Mom 9:00	Inner: no symbols	Inner: School 9:00

Table 8.7 Step six, size and distance, Example 8.A

Male: dark blue	Female: light blue	MS1: green	MS2: orange	FS: brown	FD: purple
Size: largest symbol is move- others are small	Size: largest stress is PA others are small	Size: symbols are large	Size: symbols are small; largest is move symbol	Size: symbols small	Size: symbols are small
Distance: CF 1 cm Move 12 cm Mother 3 cm	Distance: Move 0.1 cm Pa 12.5 cm CS 4.5 cm	Distance: no distance symbols touch his symbol	Distance: Mom 2.5 cm School 4 cm Soccer 0.3 cm Move 8.2 cm	Distance: School 11.7 cm Soccer 11.8 cm Move 1.5 cm	Distance: Boys 3.5 cm School 1.2 cm

are not as much of a concern. The stress symbol about school and sports appear to be not so significant. Female son has his school and sports stresses at some distance indicating that he does not experiences them as intensely. The younger children place small stresses for school and sports but place small symbols that are close to their own symbol.

Children placing symbols in the FLSD will often be concerned about the situations that affect their everyday life. We often see stress symbols drawn by siblings about their siblings and it would seem that this is not a huge concern by its placement in the lower section of the drawing. However, since it was placed on the drawing it needs to be investigated as to whatever issues the symbol represents to the daughter.

The children express some mixed messages on the move. The youngest son places the move stress far away from him in a zone that indicates it is not so significant to him. The female's son placed the stress for move just above the 9:00 region. The symbol is his largest for stress but it is located in the outer zone and in a position of close proximity to his own position. The male's oldest son places the symbol for move stress in a large and significant location next to himself and his mother. The close proximity and high placement indicate some concern.

The male's oldest son demonstrates the most concern with the placement of his stress symbols. The symbols take up most of the space in the outer and middle zone by the 1:00 region. The symbol indicates some serious stress related to the move and the impact that move will have on his mother. The therapist can reflect back to this symbol placement either in the process of conducting the drawing or refer back to it when working on treatment plans. The male's children have each placed a symbol of concern for their mother. Referencing both symbols can spread the pressure off the oldest son and indicate that both are concerned about Mom in order to gain more information about how this concern affects each of them.

The male's oldest son indicates through his symbol size and placements that he has the most emotional connection to his stress and it indicates an area of concern for this family. He appears in this drawing to be in the middle of divided loyalties between his parents. Observe the placement with both parents at opposite sides of the 10:00 and 2:00 regions and the son is in the middle. He also has a strong sense of self with the possibility that he has been given too much power in his role as oldest son above all other immediate family members. He is in a separate place in this family symbol with most of the other family members located on the left side of the drawing away from him. His closest family member in this drawing is his father with both of them located in the upper middle zone. This placement information can be used in a positive manner by encouraging both the female son and the male son 1 to take leadership in an age appropriate way. It would be important to be mindful of being sensitive in this issue to avoid causing stress to the male son 1's role where he already shares a serious stress about his mother.

The adults were able to indicate how they might be feeling about the move and children's adjustment. The male in this family expresses a small concern about the children fighting and places it close to emotional center. He reports that the children usually get along well but it bothers him when the children squabble. While he has a large symbol for the move he places the symbol in the outer zone in a high placement possibly indicating that the move is considered manageable, important, and low on his stress level. The placement and size of this symbol and the meaning the male applies to it need to be investigated. The other stress symbols show that they are important to him as he places them closest to him but also in smaller size. In the adult male's discussion, he expresses a concern about his mother but states that it is an ongoing everyday stress. Once again, these symbols indicate that he is managing the stress. The location and size of the stress symbols have to be considered in order to obtain some insights as to the meaning of the symbol. In this instance, the size counters the location and vice versa. If the lower location also included a smaller symbol it might indicate a lesser concern. A larger symbol such as the one placed in the inner zone reveals his concern for children and a significant location of emotional concern.

The female's symbols reveal a move stress symbol that is close to her symbol connected to changing her living arrangements. She also places in this drawing a symbol of concern about sharing parenting with her stepchildren's mother without making negative comments to the children. She places her largest stress symbol next to the symbol for children's mother and makes a statement to the facilitator about her concern. This is one of the values of the symbolic drawing that it indicates clues as to what is going on for clients in a visual way. Any concerns about parenting can be explored in private sessions.

STEP EIGHT: COMMUNICATION LINES

Male Adult

Spouse: good
Son1: good
Son2: good
Mother: so-so
Father: so-so
Sister: good
Stepson: good
Stepdaughter: good
Ex-wife: poor
Pet: so-so
Work: good
Running: good
Children's school: good
Children's activities: good
Spiritual practice: poor
Move: good
Children fighting: so-so
Mother stress: so-so

Adult Female

Spouse: good
Son: good
Daughter: good
Mother: good
Father: good
Brother: so-so
Stepson 1: so-so
Stepson 2: good
Ex-husband: good
Pet: good
Work: good
Exercise: good
Children's school: good
Children's activities: good
Move: good
Children's school: good
Parenting: so-so

Adult Female's son

Mother: good
Father: good
Stepfather: good
Uncle: so-so
Sister: good
Maternal grandmother: good
Maternal grandfather: good
Paternal grandmother: good
Paternal grandfather: good
Stepbrother 1: good
Stepbrother 2: good
School: good
Soccer: good
Dad's house: good
Changing school: good
New soccer team: so-so
Move: so-so

Adult Female's daughter

Mother: good
Father: good
Brother: good
Stepfather: good
Uncle: so-so
Maternal grandmother: good
Maternal grandfather: good
Paternal grandmother: good
Paternal grandmother: good
Stepbrother 1: so-so
Stepbrother 2 so-so

Pet: good
School: good
Dance: good
New school: so-so
Boys' things: poor

Adult Male's Son 1

Mother: good
Father: good
Paternal grandfather: good
Paternal grandmother: good
Aunt: good
Maternal grandmother: so-so
Maternal grandfather: so-so
Stepbrother: good
Stepsister: so-so
Pet: good
Mom's house: good
School: good
Soccer: good
Mom alone: poor
Move: good

Adult Male's son 2

Mother: good
Father: good
Stepmother: good
Brother: good
Paternal grandmother: good
Paternal grandfather: good
Maternal grandmother: so-so
Maternal grandfather: so-so
Aunt: good
Stepbrother: good
Stepsister: so-so
Pet: good
School: good
Soccer: good
Mom alone: poor
Move: good
Sharing with stepsister: poor

Reflections on Step Eight: Family Case Example 8.A

These lines confirm the messages placed in the drawing as far as the symbols and their placements being managed by this family. The lines of poor communication relate to stressors. There is a so-so connection between the male's oldest son and the stepmother. The oldest son expressed a concern that his mother would not like it if he was too friendly with his new stepmother. Other so-so communication lines indicate communication issues with other relatives which might require some more questioning as to the meaning of the quality of the communication.

Using the FLSD With Family Case Example 8.A

This drawing creates an opportunity to ask the children about the symbols they placed on the drawing and begin to find out more information about the visual placements. Questions related to the symbols such as noticing that the male's son 1 seems all out by himself is an opportunity to see if the family or the child has any concern about that situation.

This drawing also creates a graphic image that provides information to the adults indicating that the children seem to be handling issues with the move in a positive way. All the children drew good communication lines to stresses related to moving. The therapist/counselor can ask questions about those communication lines and let the children expand on what those lines mean to them. We would make assumptions that the good communication lines mean they are OK about the move. That being said it is always good to check that assumption out with family members. The drawing also shows some other strengths related to coping with stress and environmental factors. This drawing is a good reference point to proceed with that discussion.

The drawing also allows for a discussion about the children's concern for their mother since two of the male's sons drew that concern. Even if the older son expresses a more intense concern in the drawing, he does not get singled out because both have drawn it. The family can then talk about ways to reassure the children and support them in coping with that stress. It would be helpful to encourage the parents validate the two son's concerns and reassure the children about the male and female's own positions of support for the male's son's love for their mother.

The drawing also can start the conversation about family strengths. The therapist can observe that the family does not appear to have many stresses and that they seem so small. Once again, any observation made by the therapist needs to be checked out with the family members to ascertain if the observer is getting the correct message from the drawing. The conversation continues no matter if the family agrees or offers a counter point in regards to the drawing.

Observing that most of the family is on the left side of the drawing and that family has very little in the way of inner zone placements begins the discussion about family goals and desires for the future evolution of this family group. Useful questions connected to the drawing point to the picture and ask the family what they see and if they would like to work toward making it different?

The drawing also is a launch pad for observing other issues with the family. Family members can express agreement or disagreement with observations made by the therapist and other family members.

Family Case Example 8.B

The following FLSD example is of an intact family experiencing a child having problems in school. The high school student is having problems with his grades and skipping school. Mom sought out counseling to help the son with the school situation. A systems-oriented counselor invited the whole family in to an assessment session to see what is happening with the whole family in order to see the best way to help the student.

The family members in this drawing include Mom, a Caucasian American of northern European descent and her husband a Caucasian American of northern European descent. This couple are in their late forties. Both of the parents work outside the home. The couple married when they were very young and had a son early in the relationship. Their oldest son is 21 years old and married, currently serving in the military. The couple have three additional children born a few years after the oldest son. Son 2, age 15 is the child in the family having

FAMILY LIFE SPACE DRAWING WITH FAMILIES | 141

trouble with school grades and behavior. Son 3, age 12 is in middle school and the youngest child a daughter age 10 is in 5th grade.

This drawing illustrates an example of how different family members can demonstrate different sizes of symbols and different experiences of family members. This is important to keep in mind as the process of the drawing evolves. Family members draw themselves when completing the family drawing but do not usually draw in other family members who are currently in the room. This drawing includes a family member who is not present and gives an example of how the various family members experience that missing member of the family. This drawing also illustrates how the focus of concern can shift from not just the person with the presenting problem but to areas of concern within the family system.

STEP THREE: PLACEMENT OF SYMBOLS OF SELF

Key to Symbols

M: Mother, orange   Son3, green   Son2, light blue
D: father, dark blue   Daughter, red

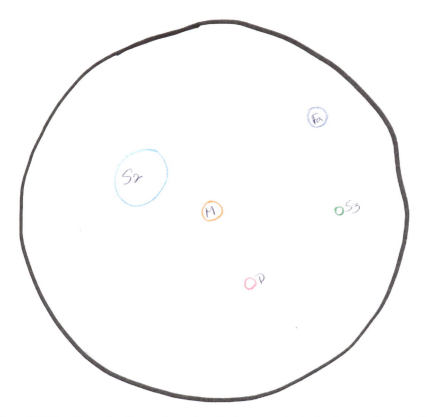

Figure 8.5 Step three, family members place their own symbols: family case, Example 8.B

Table 8.8 Step three: placement of symbols for family members, Example 8.B

Mom: orange	Father: dark blue	Son2: light blue	Son3: green	Daughter: red
Location: in the center of the inner zone in the 12:00–6:00 region	Location: Outer zone, 2:00 region	Location: Inner and middle zone, covering 10:00 and 9:00 region	Middle zone 3:00 region	Location; lower inner zone slightly left of 6:00
Size: Slightly on small size	Slightly larger than mother's symbol	Extra-large symbol compared to others	Extra-small symbol	Small symbol

Reflections on Step Three: Family Case Example 8.B

This family drawing has all the family members spread out over the family symbol. Family members seem to be in isolated sections of the drawing. The mother and daughter are in the inner zone reflecting an emotional connection to the heart of the family. Healthy family functioning would show both parents in the inner zone. In this family drawing the father is out in the outer zone, almost in a position that suggests he is disengaging from the family.

Son 2 has an extra-large symbol compared to other family members and it reflects either an inflated sense of self or an indication that he has too much power that might be affecting this family. His symbol is positioned partially in the inner and middle zone is off to the left of this zone in a space alone by himself.

The symbol and placement of Son 3 indicates that he is also isolated in the middle zone in a very small symbol. A symbol of this size often indicates a low sense of esteem or a sense that the person might feel that they are not too important. He is not the lowest symbol in this family so it may be an indication of other factors. The daughter's symbol is also small located in the inner zone and is the lowest positioned member of this family.

STEP FOUR: SIGNIFICANT OTHERS

This drawing continues the interaction with family members by having each person come to drawing board and add other people that are not in the room but important to the family. In this situation, the family has an older brother and a sister-in-law. Everyone in the family added the brother but not everyone added the sister-in-law. The people in the family are asked to place people that they feel are like family. In this family, we ask about parents of the parents and whether or not they have siblings. In the course of completing the drawing we ask about the parents to determine if they are living we ask about where they live currently and is this place where the adult client grew up. In cases where the parent may have died we asked about the circumstances of the parental death. It is important to learn about how old the client was at the time of parental death and if the parent experienced a prolonged illness. In this family, we learn that the mother's parents are currently living and that the family lives several states away. The parents live in the same home in which the woman grew up. The mother in this family has one sibling who lives in another region of the country and that she does have much contact with him. The father in this family informs us that his mother and father divorced when he was a young man. His father remarried but is currently deceased. His mother never remarried and lives several hours away. The father's widow also lives several hours away. He has one sister who lives nearby and she has a family that interacts with his family.

FAMILY LIFE SPACE DRAWING WITH FAMILIES | 143

Key to Symbols

FA: Father, dark blue

FM: father's mother
FF: father's father
S: sister
S1: son 1
SW: son's wife
SM: stepmother

Son 2: light blue

B1: brother 1
A: aunt
U: uncle
P: pet
MGM: maternal grandmother
MGF: maternal grandfather
PGM: paternal grandmother

U-Uncle
A-Aunt
MGM-Maternal grandmother
MGF: maternal grandfather

M: Mother, orange

MM: mother's mother
MF: mother's father
B: brother
S1: son 1
SW: son's wife

Son 3: green

B1: brother 1
A: aunt
U: uncle
P: pet
MGM: maternal grandmother
MGF: maternal grandfather
PGF: paternal grandfather
FR: friend

Daughter: red

PGM: paternal grandmother Fr: friend
PGF: paternal grandfather
B1: brother 1
P: pet

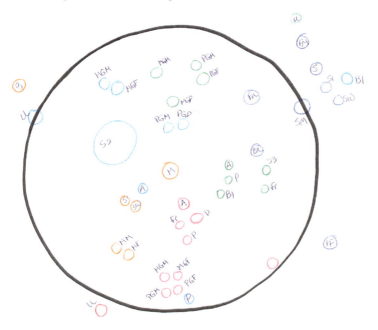

Figure 8.6 Step four, placement of significant others: family case, Example 8.B

Table 8.9 Step four, significant others: zone and region, Example 8.B

Mom: orange	Dad: dark blue	Son2: light blue	Son3: green	Daughter: red
Outside: Brother 10:00	Outside: Mother 2:00, father 4:00, sister 2:00, Son1 2:00 Son's wife 2:00 Stepmother 2:00	Outside-Brother 1 2:00 Uncle 10:00 partial	Outside: Uncle 1:00 region	Outside: Uncle between 6:00 and 7:00
Outer: Zero	Outer: stepmother between this zone and outside at 2:00	Outer: Uncle on the edge of outside and outer 10:00, MGM at 11:00 lower edge of outer, Pet at 6:00	Outer: PGM close to 12:00, MGM partially outer and middle zone 11:00	Outer: MGM, MGF, PGF PGM 6:00 region, Brother 1–4 5:00 region
Middle: Mother and father 7:00 region	Middle: brother-in-law close to 3:00	MGF 11:00	Middle: friend below 3:00 MGF on edge of inner close to 12:00, PGF near PGM at 12:00	Middle: Pet near 6:00
Inner: Son1 and his wife near 8:00 region	Inner: no symbols	Inner: aunt at 8:00, PGM and PGF at 12:00	Inner: B1 lower edge at 4:00 region, aunt close to edge of inner at 3:00, pet 3:00	Inner: aunt close to 6:00 region Pet 6:00

Table 8.10 Step four: size and distance, Example 8.B

	Mom: orange	Dad: dark blue	Son2: light blue	Son3: green	Daughter: red
size	These symbols are similar to her own symbol size. The smallest is for her son's wife	Symbols are similar in size His largest symbol is for his mother	His symbol is the largest on the drawing. Others are on the small size	Symbol for self is extra small. Others are small	Symbols on the small size largest symbol for uncle.
Distance	Son1 2.5 cm Son's wife 2.5 cm Brother 9 cm Mother 5 cm Father 5 cm	Brother-in-law 2.4 cm Stepmother 1.1 cm Father 9.8 cm Mother 2.5 cm Sister 1.5 cm Son1 2 cm Wife 6.4 cm	Uncle 3 cm MGM 1.5 cm MGF 1.4 cm PGM 2.1 cm PGF 1.9 cm Aunt 3 cm Pet 9.7 cm Brother1 10.1 cm	Uncle 10 cm Aunt 1.9 MGF 8 cm MGM 9.5 cm PGF 8 cm PGM 8.5 cm Brother1 2.6 cm	Aunt 1 cm Brother1 4.2 cm Friend 1 cm Pet 1.5 cm MGM 4.4 cm MGF 3.8 cm PGF 4.5 cm PGM 4.8 cm

Reflections on Step Four: Family Case Example 8.B

The placement of significant others by each family member demonstrates how people in the same family can have a different experience of another family member. The missing oldest brother is a good example of this phenomena. Mother and Son3 included brother 1 in the inner zone. Each one of those placed Brother 1 in different regions. Mother has Son 1 near the 8:00 region and Son 3 at the 4:00 region. Mother and Son 3 see the Brother 1 in a lower region of the inner circle still a position of emotional connection. For the mother, it could be placed this way because she sees herself as hierarchically above her son in the line of emotional responsibility and authority in this family. Son 3 may also recognize this position.

The daughter sees brother 1 in lower regions of the symbol in the outer zone. This could possibly due to the fact they have a large age difference and she has not been around this brother in a long time and did not have a lot of connection with him. This placement could also be reflective of her own difficult sense of the role the brother placed in the family.

Father places Son1 in a high position but outside the family. The high position reflects that father connects a sense of significance to his son but his placement outside the family symbol indicates a disconnect. Son2 also places his older brother in the region of his father's symbols outside at 2:00 a position that recognizes respect but includes a disconnect.

Most of father's symbols are outside the family symbol which causes concern that he might not think these people belong in the family or that he himself might be making plans to leave this family and take others with him. The location of these placements close to his own symbol do reflect that he is close to these significant others but sees them outside this family symbol. The distance between his symbol and the connection to the family symbol suggests a potential for the father leaving the family as it currently stands. These placements are important to investigate and do indicate an area of concern.

The mother's symbols in this drawing reveal a possible disconnect with her family of origin by viewing her symbol for her brother outside the family symbol and her parents in a low section of the family symbol. It could potentially be useful to explore these placements and attempt to understand family attachment issues. Mother does indicate that she is in the emotional center of this family.

It is interesting to note that some family members like Son3 place significant others in upper regions of the symbols and other family members such as the daughter place every symbol in the lower regions. Lower regions usually indicate some self-esteem or low positions of power in family drawings. These positional placements indicate different experiences and emotional sense of the same people.

STEP FIVE: ENVIRONMENTAL SYMBOLS

Step five has each family member to come to the drawing board again and place symbols that reflect places and activities that affect them and the family. These activities are labeled environmental factors.

In the course of completing this drawing we learn that the mother in this family has employment as a book keeper outside the home. She places symbols for her children's school and symbols for church and a separate symbol for Jesus. While she also places a symbol for her husband's work she lets us know that she has some difficult feelings about it.

The husband also places symbols for work and indicates that he has employment outside the home but also has a side business. He places symbols for his children's school and church. These symbols also get placed on the outside of the family symbol.

Son2 has symbols for his parents work and only has two other symbols for school and church. Son3 places symbols for school and youth group, church. The daughter places symbols for her parents work and church along with a symbol for school.

The process of completing environmental factors allows the therapist to learn about activities that the family engages in on a regular basis. The therapist asks questions about the activities as they interact with each client when they have a turn at the board. This is a crucial component of joining with each person in the family individually.

The following chart lists the various activities of each family member and describes the placements of the environmental symbols in the various zones and regions of the family symbol. The next chart identifies size and distance.

Key to Symbols

Mother: orange

MW: Mom's work
Dw: Dad's work
C: Church
S: School
J: Jesus

Son2: light blue

DW: Dad's work
MW: Mom's work
C: church
S: school
H: House

S: school
Church: church
SH: shopping

Father: dark blue

W1: Main employment
W2: side business
C: Church
J: Jesus
S: children's school

Son3: green

Church
Youth group
DW: Dad's work
MW: Mom's work
S: school

Daughter: red

DW: Dad's work
Mw: Mom's work

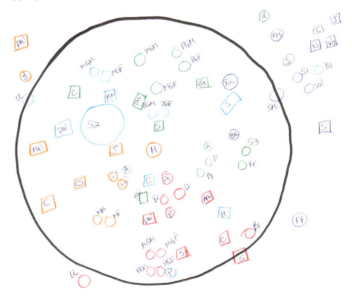

Figure 8.7 Step five, environmental symbols: family case, Example 8.B

Table 8.11 Step five, environmental symbols: zones and regions, Example 8.B

Mom: orange	Dad: dark blue	Son2: light blue	Son3: green	Daughter: red
Outside: Dad's work far corner at 11:00 region	Outside: Far edges of paper in the 2:00 region, Work 1 and 2 church Jesus At 3:00 he places school in the outside region of symbol	Outside: no placements	Outside: No symbols	Outside: partial outside shopping at 5:00
Outer: Church 8:00 region	No symbols	Outer: Dad's work some in middle zone, partially in outer At 9:00 School partially 2:00 House partially in outer and middle 5:00	Outer: Church at 10:00	Outer: Church 5:00–6:00 School 6:00
Middle Children's school 8:00 region	Middle: no symbols	Middle: corner of Dad's work at 9:00 Corner of school at 2:00 Corner of house 5:00	Middle: a corner of Church at 10:00 Youth group 1:00 Corner of Dad's work 12:00	Middle: Dad's work 6:00 Mom's work 5:00
Inner: Jesus 9:00	Inner: no symbols	Inner: church at 6:00	Inner: Dad's work 12:00 School 12:00 Mom's work 6:00	Inner: no symbols

Table 8.12 Step five, environmental symbols: size and distance, Example 8.B

Mom: orange	Dad: dark blue	Son2: light blue	Son3: green	Daughter: red
Size: her symbols are similar in size with exception of Dad's work	Size: similar in size; considered small	Size: largest symbol Dad's work; House smallest symbol Others are similar in size to each other	Size: symbols are small but largest Is symbol for church; smallest symbol Mom's work	Size: symbols are similar to each other
Distance: Mom's work 5.2 cm Dad's work 11.5 cm Church 6.7 cm School 5 cm Jesus 0.7 cm	Distance: Work1 4.2 cm Work2 5.2 cm Church 5.5 cm School 3.6 cm Jesus 6.5 cm	Distance: School 5 cm House 8.2 cm Church 4.2 cm Dad's work 1 cm Mom's work 0.5 cm	Distance: School 3.7 cm Youth group 6.6 cm Church 11.7 cm Mom's work 7.3 cm Dad's work 7 cm	Distance: School 3 cm Church 3 cm Shopping 4.4 cm Dad's work 2.5 cm Mom's work 2.5 cm

Reflections on Step Five: Family Case Example 8.B

According to Mostwin (1980), symbols placed in the upper half of the family symbol have high regard and symbols placed low in the family symbol have low regard. Each person creates their own frame of reference by placing themselves in the drawing. Sometimes a person will follow the upper and lower process indicating their own regard for symbols connected to them. For example, in this drawing we see the Father with his symbols outside the family symbol but he still demonstrates a sense of regard for where he places these symbols in the 2:00 section of the outside family region. Symbols in the higher regions indicate respect and vice versa. If we follow the premise that distance between the symbol for self and environmental symbol indicates a sense of emotional closeness (Barker & Barker, 1990) we can learn more about the family member's connections to the environmental components.

Symbols placed for Dad's work are closer to Son2 and the daughter than the symbol that the father placed for his own work. Dad saw his work at 4.2 cm and 5.2 cm near him. Son2 placed Dad's work at 0.1 cm near his own symbol. The youngest child, the daughter also placed Dad's work close to her at 2.5 cm near her symbol.

Other family members placed Dad's work much more distant from their own symbols. The mother's symbol for Dad's work was the most distant and outside the family symbol, but also fairly large and in a place of high regard. Son 3 also placed Dad's work in a position of high regard but distant from himself. These symbol placements indicate that the mother most likely has some disconnects about her husband's work but values what it provides. The Son2 placements may be reinforcing concerns that he is stepping into a caretaker role in the family and feeling a burden of responsibility. Being overly responsible is an inappropriate role for him and may be the source of school issues. He feels closer to the parents work than the parents apparently seem to feel.

Other observations relate to the symbol for church. While all family members placed church on the drawing some see church in a lesser place than others. Even the mother who has a symbol for Jesus (her faith) above her own symbol places church itself in a distant place of lesser regard. This leads us to make assumption that she does not like her church but feels close to her Christian faith. Father places church and Jesus in a place of high regard but demonstrates his greatest distance from both. Son3 seems to have the least emotional connection to church than the other children as evidenced by his distance from the symbol. He places the symbol in high regard at the 10:00 region but distant from his own symbol. These symbolic representations open the door for asking questions about these very thoughts and assumptions. The placement of symbols and the distance and size of the symbol are opportunities for investigating the meaning applied to each symbol placed by each person in the family. An example would be asking the Mother about her church. "I see your faith is important to you what's going on at your church? Are you unhappy there?"

Step Six: Stress Symbols

The next phase of completing the FLSD involves asking the family members to include a symbol for stresses that might be affecting each person. The concept of stress is also referenced as something that might be a concern or worry including something positive in your life such as being a good parent or doing a good job in school.

In this drawing, the family did not list a large number of concerns. The mother had the most concerns and she identified them as worries for her extended family that does not live near her. She also expressed concern about politics and people who have different political concerns than her own beliefs. She expressed a stress about housework and her children. She also listed a stress symbol for her husband's work and for money issues. Symbols for financial concerns is a commonly drawn stress symbol in the FLSD.

FAMILY LIFE SPACE DRAWING WITH FAMILIES

The father symbolized concerns for his work and money as well as a worry about Son1 who is in the military and stationed far away. He stated that these were his main concerns. He places these symbols near his other symbols.

Son2 symbolized his only stress as school and Son3 joined his brother in symbolizing a stress for school. Son3 added stress symbols for his grandmother, who he said was sick recently and also added a symbol for his sister getting into his things at home. The daughter only had two stress symbols for kids at school teasing her and a worry about a family at church who was having trouble and needed prayers.

The following chart illustrates the stress symbol and their placements in the various zone of the family drawing. An additional chart follows that lists observations on size and distance.

Key to Symbols

Mother: orange

EF: extended family
Politics
H: House
S: Son
B: Business
$: money
c: children

Father: dark blue

W1: Work one
W2: Work two
$: money
S1: Son 1

Son2: light blue

S: School

Son3: green

S: School
GM: Grandmother
S: Sister

Daughter: red

Kids at school
Family at church

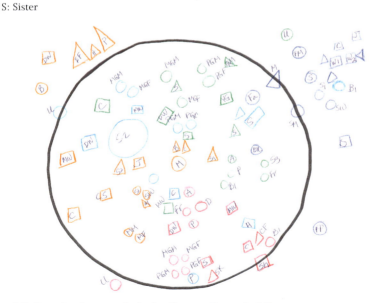

Figure 8.8 Step six, stress symbols: family case, Example 8.B

Table 8.13 Step six, stress symbols: zone and region, Example 8.B

Mother: orange	Dad: dark blue	Son2: light blue	Son3: green	Daughter: red
Outside: no placements	Work 2 2:00 Son1 2:00 Money partial outside 2:00 Work1 2:00	Outside: no symbols	Outside: no symbols	Outside: no symbols
Outer: 11:00 extended family Politics housework	Outer Most of money in 2:00	Outer: no symbols	Outer: GM 1:00	Outer: Kids at school 6:00 Family at church 5:00
Middle: son2 3:00 partially in inner zone	Middle: no symbols	Middle: School 2:00	Middle: Sister 12:00 School 2:00	Middle: no symbols
Inner: Son1 3:00 Money 7:00 Business 12:00 Children 12:00	Inner: no symbols	Inner: no symbols	Inner: no symbols	Inner: no symbols

Table 8.14 Step six, stress symbols: size and distance, Example 8.B

Mother: orange	Father: dark blue	Son2: light blue	Son3: green	Daughter: red
Size: large symbols outside Large for sons	Size: largest is for work 1; the rest are small	Size: smaller than his own symbol	Size: larger than his own symbol	Size: similar to other symbol size
Distance: Extended family 9.5 cm Politics 8.7 cm Housework 7.5 cm Children 0.4 cm Money 3.2 cm Son2 3.5 cm Son1 1.5 cm	Distance: Work1 4.3 cm Work2 5.8 cm Money 0.5 cm Son1 3 cm	Distance: School 5 cm	Distance: School 3.8 cm Grandma 10.6 cm Sister 8.5 cm	Distance: Kids at school 4 cm Church family 3.3 cm

Reflections on Step Six: Family Case Example 8.B

Stress symbols are for the most part located outside the family center, indicating that the stressors are not a particular pressure in this family. Mother has placed three stress symbols in the center but they are small symbols with the exception of Son1 in this section of the inner circle. The symbols with the highest regard are distant from her and we would assume that she does not have much connection to these stresses even though they are held in a highly regarded position. Son 3 places three stress symbols in the middle zone. Most of the stress in this family for other family members is located outside the family symbol or on its edges.

Most of these symbols do not reflect a large size in the family drawing but it is noted that the Mother has five stress symbols in or near the inner zone. Her largest symbols are for concerns about her two older sons. The mother has the most symbols and her closest emotional connection to the symbols would be concerned with the children at 0.4 cm. The father's closest concern is money and work. The children have few stresses and those that they do have are symbolized at a relative distance from their own symbol. Family members who placed symbols in highly regarded places have also sometimes placed them at a distance from their own symbol. The father has been consistent in placing his symbols closest to him which shows he has some close connection to the symbols he has drawn.

USING THE FLSD WITH FAMILY CASE EXAMPLE 8.B

This family indicates that some family members such as Son 2 see themselves as very large and some people such as Son 3 see themselves as very small. The parent's symbols are very separated in this drawing and the Father is located away from the inner zone. All of his symbols are located outside the family symbol. With the exception of the symbol for finances located partially in the outer zone. When reviewing this drawing with the family it would be useful to point out these observations and ask people what they think about these placements and symbols. Any observation by other family members need to be heard and validated by the therapist.

In this family, the original presenting concern was connected to the mother's concern for the behavior and performance of Son 2 in school. When the family completed the FLSD, the mother expressed concern about what she saw in the family drawing. She was surprised that the family member's symbols were in separate places all over the symbol. The mother also expressed concerned about Son 3 and his placement in a small symbol toward the outer edge of the family.

The father of the family also expressed concern that he was mostly on the outside of the family drawing. The parents decided to revise their original concern and do some work together to help their children. They were concerned that the problem in the family might have more to do with their own relationship versus the son having school problems. They wanted to learn to work together better in an effort to help their children.

The visual nature of this demonstration helped everyone to see how family members might experience themselves in this family. Everyone observed the isolation and the adults noticed how far apart they were. The FLSD was able to demonstrate the family situation to this family and expand the area of original concern to a broader more systemic observation. The visual aspect of seeing the placements spoke volumes to the parents and helped them to identify the areas of concern for therapeutic intervention.

SUMMARY: FLSD WITH FAMILIES

Meeting families to engage in family treatment can be a complicated task as the therapist attempts to uncover the multiple layers of treatment considerations and concerns. Participating in the process of the FLSD allows family members to evaluate their situation from a perspective that includes all the family members and will give them a holistic picture of the family situation. The interactive expressive nature of the process has family members looking on with deep interest to see where others in the family group might place their symbols and what they each might identify throughout all the steps along the way. Usually family members report that they enjoy completing the process.

As each family is unique and presents with individual components so will the various FLSDs that will emerge as the therapists and counselors begins to explore using this process. The FLSD will offer potential unique layers of information that might never have been expressed in a regular counseling session. The individual expression of each family member placing symbols in same space of the drawing creates an image that helps the family literally be seen in the beginning of the treatment process.

References

Barker, S. B., & Barker, R. T. (1990). Investigation of the construct validity of the family life space diagram. *Journal of Mental Health Counseling*, 2(4), 506–514.

Mostwin, D. (1980). *Social dimension of family treatment*. Washington, DC: National Association of Social Workers.

CHAPTER NINE
Family Life Space Drawing (FLSD) in Various Counseling Settings

FLSD IN VARIOUS COUNSELING SETTINGS

Focusing on finding ways to help troubled families facing modern family crises was the creative force behind the development of the FLSD. Mostwin (1980a) developed the graphic expressive process of the FLSD as a way to first understand the basic makeup of a family situation and to obtain unspoken messages about family dynamics. Mostwin was excited about the ecological concepts of understanding the human condition beyond the individual perspective that was popular in the psychological training of her educational time frame. She embraced systemic concepts and viewed family assessment as an exploration of the family life space that went beyond the nuclear family and extended family to incorporate environmental and psychological factors. Dr. Mostwin promoted family therapy as a way to help families cope with the changing patterns of a post-WWII society (Mostwin, 1980b). The concern for challenges to the traditional functions of the family made her a strong proponent of developing a treatment model for families and troubled youth. Incorporating the FLSD a way to assess families in the beginning sessions of treating at-risk youth she created treatment teams providing intensive interventions for clients and trainings for student interns. Upon leaving the training centers and teaching clinics, student interns took the FLSD expressive process and applied it to various settings of social work and mental health practice.

Some of the work settings involved, social services agencies, mental health centers, schools, psychiatric facilities, nursing homes, substance abuse settings, and agencies serving children in need of intensive family treatment. This chapter provides examples of using the FLSD in various settings and explores some of the unique aspects of the process and interventions that facilitate and enhance basic mental health and life functioning.

The FLSD is offered as a qualitative assessment method that mostly facilitates the development of the client therapist relationship. We offer that the interactive nature of the FLSD provides the client with the valuable therapeutic engagement process so necessary to future treatment. Patterson, Williams, Edwards, Chamow, and Grauf-Grounds (2009) state that the joining process is enhanced when clients have a chance to tell their story and feel heard and understood. The FLSD can adapt to any model or theory of treatment. It does not have to be restricted to its original intent of the STMFI.

Following a qualitative assessment process does not necessarily create a defined pattern of measurement for developing assessment markers in the way that standardized measures offer.

Even so, the qualitative process of the FLSD has an advantage over quantitative standardized measures in that it is client specific. Standardized assessment measures have some limitations in actual clinical settings as therapists are reluctant to utilized them, considering the measures not relevant to the actual work of marriage and family therapy (Lavee & Avisar, 2006). A potential issue connected to not using standardized measures might be connected to therapists not actually being adequately trained in the methods of quantitative assessment (Deacon & Piercy, 2001, pp. 357–358). Research from Israel by Lavee and Avisar (2006) discovered that only 27.6% of marriage and family therapists use standardized assessments with school social workers more likely than psychologists to use standardized assessments measures. With the possibilities of these considerations Deacon and Piercy (2001) offer that the current focus on constructionist thought favors the qualitative method of family assessment in that it offers client specific meaning to families and therapists. The FLSD favors the situational assessment and client specific approach to meeting and evaluating families and couples in the first session.

The FLSD has the ability to adapt to any counseling setting and therapeutic model related to systems theory. The authors have utilized this process when working from almost every orientation of family therapy intervention. We have applied this process in opening sessions of family therapy when operating from structural, strategic, solution-focused, and problem-solving approaches. We have utilized this assessment process in our work as couple's counselors operating as Imago therapists, and emotionally focused couples counseling.

This chapter will share examples of using the FLSD in various counseling settings that we as clinical social workers have previous knowledge and experience in observing the FLSD applied in initial sessions. This chapter will share examples of using the FLSD in social service agencies and psychiatric facilities as well as a school setting. The cases include a foster care situation focusing on consideration of termination of parental rights, working with a severely psychotic family member in a psychiatric facility, and with a school working with deaf students. This chapter will also provide a brief discussion about use in other settings.

These applications of utilizing the FLSD will demonstrate its ability to help families focus on issues that would not be verbalized or apparent without the symbolic process. The following examples are composite situations drawn from our past knowledge of other professional and our vast experience in different mental health settings. Many of specific details have been changed to protect identity of clients but the exciting outcomes of using the FLSD are true.

Social Service Settings

Social service agencies provide services to many different types of populations and programs. The FLSD has been used in a variety of social service settings to assist with the process of determining client services and for providing interventions intended to help remediate problem states. Social service agencies can work with children and protective service, additionally these agencies provide foster care and adoption services. Other programs in social or family service agencies support programs to help the elderly. In addition to providing support and protection to populations unable to advocate for themselves, family service agencies help people experiencing the detrimental effects of poverty.

Foster Care and Adoption

Social service agencies that work with foster care children and families have used the FLSD to help provide direction in developing treatment plans for children involved with the agency. Protective service workers have used the process to assist and support families and children under stress by exploring the meaning of symbols placed in the drawing related to family members and environment, and psychological stress issues. This process is especially useful for children who might be hesitant to verbally express a concern but will symbolically represent an issue or concern through the placement of symbols.

Social service agencies who look to provide older children with adoption placement can use the FLSD process to investigate unspoken concerns about past family of origin and future hesitations about adoptive or foster families. The symbolic placement of family members can potentially report on a sense of emotional closeness or distance for the person drawing the symbols. A child might indicate that they do not care about a biological parent but the FLSD could indicate that the person is closer to the child if they place the symbol for that biological parent in the inner zone of their drawing or closer to their own symbol. Barker, Barker, Dawson, and Knisely (1997) discovered that symbols drawn for a human or pet indicated support when they were drawn close to the person's own symbol. It is a common experience in using this process with clients to hear children and adults report that they had no intention of saying anything before the counseling interview only to find themselves sharing a great deal of information in the process of the drawing.

The FLSD is an excellent starting tool for interviewing prospective adoptive parents. The FLSD reveals family of origin issues and identifies strengths and areas of need for people considering adoption. Clients considering adoption can add a symbol for future adoption on the drawing. The placement and size of the symbols has the potential to provide unspoken information about the preadoption experience. Counselors have used the drawing as a way to engage in preadoption evaluation and preparation by discussing placements and talking about the various symbols placed in the drawing.

Supporting People in Poverty

Social workers working with people experiencing poverty can use the FLSD to investigate the unspoken experience of living with limited resources. The information gathered from the symbolic representations can be utilized as starting points for guiding the conversation toward client desires and treatment goals. The FLSD has clients draw family members but also environmental and social symbols that report on involvement or lack of involvement with community resources. Symbolic placements can often begin to share about the experience of working with those community resources in ways that words would not be able to convey. An example might pertain to negative experiences with a specific housing program. The housing program might be placed in a lower position outside the family symbol with accompanying so-so or poor communication lines. This visual representation might be indicating some systemic issues with the program or some other involvement with this program. As the counselor explores and makes up conjectures about the symbol size and placements, these conjectures can be offered to the client for their consideration and discussion. Many times, clients will be hesitant to voice concerns but will illustrate them through the process of the symbolic drawing. Counselors will take cues from the placements and ask questions about the client's experience and thought processes related to the drawing and symbolic representations.

The symbolic drawing also can allude to issues and coping mechanisms related to life stress. The placing of symbols related to stress can create discussions on the management of community relief programs or point to the need for developing more resources. Regular discussion and regular interviewing are time tested and tried and true techniques of the helping profession. Adding the process of the FLSD creates a potential for discovering the unconscious dimensions that clients themselves did not even have awareness to report. Many times, counselors will point to symbols placed by clients and make observations about the symbol drawn such as it is a small or large symbol. I am wondering what it is like for you in that situation as it relates to the symbol.

Immigrants

The symbolic drawing provides another way to communicate information for people coming in for community services where the client's first language is different from the agency providing services. Italian community services worked with immigrants from three different countries and used the FLSD to gain information about relational patterns and adjustment to the new hosting community (Gennari, Tamanza, & Accordini, 2015). Clients may not have enough new language knowledge to communicate directly about issues related to adjustment distress and family connections. The symbolic nature of the drawing provides a nonverbal clue about specific difficulties that can be investigated through the use of language interpreters. For instance, an immigrant might draw a small symbol for self in a low section of the family life space. This symbolic representation might be a clue of low self-esteem or a sense of inadequacy. The symbolic placement could also be reflective of a cultural demonstration that seeks to follow a humble path. In any event, the counselor needs to follow up on all representations in order to understand the conscious or unconscious representations from each of the unique cultures that might be attempting to express some information. The FLSD is a useful tool in developing cultural competency with immigrant families. The Italian researchers discovered that the FLSD a cultural relevant expression for clients to express their own culture without interferences from the researchers own culture bias (Gennari et al., 2015).

The FLSD allows for the visual representation of information for people who do not know the right words to use as well as providing the visual representations for unconscious concerns. Counselors can view the FLSD with the client and begin to explore the meaning of the symbols with the clients. This interactive process will be most important especially when considering the assumptions made about the meaning of the symbols. Any symbolic placement needs to be investigated and that investigation can often start with the counselor's questions.

Aging Services

Social service agencies providing services for aging populations can use the FLSD as an evaluation tool to explore the intricacies and dynamics of family relationships. The process of the FLSD can identify family disconnects and strong connections. The process can help reinforce the strengths of the family or identify areas of concern that need new community resources and support. The FLSD can be utilized to review involvement with community resources as well as identifying stresses. As we have previously noted, this process is most useful when verbal skills are not as strong but can also be used effectively with highly verbal clients. The FLSD process has been used with the elderly either by conducting an individual drawing with the client to review their current situation and past. It can also be used with the elderly's whole family as a way to assess family connections and resources as a whole group.

Social service organizations have an almost infinite opportunity for application of the FLSD. The process can be used as an initial engagement tool to meet and learn about the client and the client's family. The process can also be utilized as a treatment intervention that gathers family members together to assess and plan for future treatment interventions. The process will clearly define family members, past and present, environmental and community elements involved with the client. In addition, the process identifies stresses or issues that point to service needs and areas of concern. The FLSD process has been used to help families find connection and closure when family members are experiencing the crisis of the imminent death of a loved one (Lesser, 1982). The terminally ill family member even participated in the process while bedridden.

FOSTER CARE AND TERMINATION OF PARENTAL RIGHTS: CASE EXAMPLE 9.A

While social and family service agencies assist with a myriad of community concerns the following example will demonstrate how the FLSD assisted with a situation involving foster care and consideration of the termination of parental rights for the parents. Government reports that as of 2015, over 670,000 children in the United States spent some time in foster care (Child Welfare Information Gateway, 2017) Unfortunately, even after parental rights had been legally terminated still 62,000 children were waiting to be adopted, and that children wait on average at least two years before finding permanent adoptive homes.

A social service agency had been working with two sisters who were Caucasian girls age 12 and 13, and had been in and out of foster care for the last 3 years. The girls started in foster care when they were 9 and 10 years old. Over that time frame the sisters had lived with a foster family who was interested in adopting the two girls. The foster care worker in the social service agency who also worked with the girl's biological mother was in the process of developing a permanent living plan for the girls. Part of the plan involved giving the mother the option to terminate her parental rights and allow the girls to be adopted by the foster family or follow through with a structured plan that would facilitate the safe return of the girls to the mother's custody and care.

The mother a Caucasian had a difficult history and had lost custody of older children by not being able to provide a safe environment for her family. The mother had a history of alcoholism and living in abusive relationships with men who were not related to the children. Recently the mother's life situation had improved. She was sober from alcohol for more than 6 months and had met a male partner that was also sober. Both had employment that facilitated renting a home and showing consistency in paying bills. Even with her lifestyle improvement she was anxious about regaining custody and wanted to provide a good future for her daughters. During the foster care arrangement, she had regular contact with her children.

The foster care worker decided to use the FLSD as a way to get a different understanding of the children's sense of family and the mother's commitment to regain custody. The social worker set up an evaluation session where counselors for the children and a separate counselor for the mother and her new boyfriend were present in the meeting. A FLSD was conducted with the mother and her boyfriend and the two girls as the primary people in the room. Other significant family members are represented in the drawing and are listed in this key. The following example will include step thee and four of the process. The family did complete steps four, five, and six but will not be illustrated for this discussion.

Step Three: Placement of Self

Table 9.1 Step three: placements of self, Example 9.A

Mother: red (M)	Lower edge of inner zone left of the 6:00 region
Boyfriend: black (BF)	Lower half of symbol 6:00 middle region
Sister1: orange (S1)	Lower half inner zone above right side of mother's symbol 6:00 region
Sister2: green	Lower half inner zone right of sister1's symbol left of 6:00

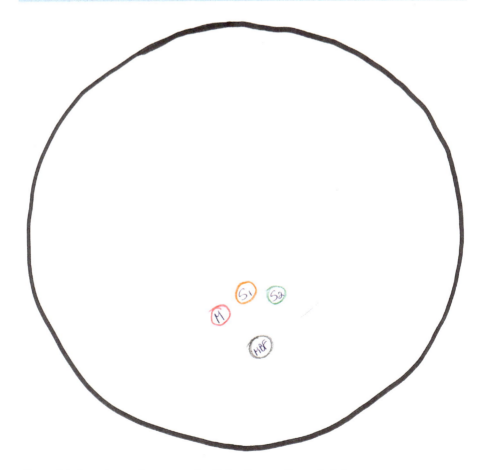

Figure 9.1 Step three, placement of self: family case, Example 9.A

STEP FOUR: PLACEMENT OF SIGNIFICANT OTHERS

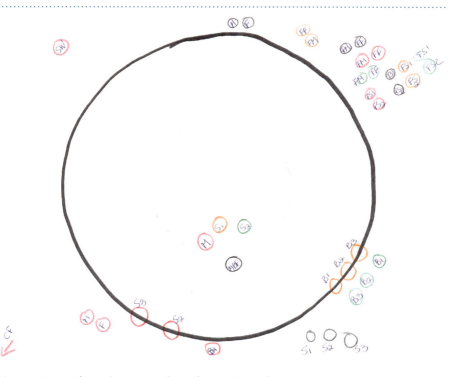

Figure 9.2 Step four, placement of significant others: family case, Example 9.A

Key to Symbols

Mother: red (M) **Boyfriend: black (BF)**

M: mother
F: father
CF: children's
B1: son 1
B2: son 2
B3: son 3
FM: foster mother
FF: foster father
FS1: foster son 1
FS2: foster son 2
SW: social worker

M: mother
F: father
father FM: foster mother
FF: foster father
FS1: foster son 1
FS2: foster son 2
B3: girlfriend (mother) son 3
B2: girlfriend (mother) son 2
B1: girlfriend (mother) son 1

Sister 1: orange **Sister 2: green**

FM: foster mother
FF: foster father

FM: foster mother
FF: foster father

FS1: foster son 1
FS2: foster Son 2
B1: brother 1
B2: brother 2
B3: brother 3

FS1: foster son 1
FS2: foster son2
B1: brother 1
B2: brother 2
B3: brother 3

Reflections on Step Four: Case Example 9.A

The family placed symbols for significant others in the family mostly outside the family symbol. The FLSD almost represents an image of "us against the world." All of the people in the room clustered their symbols in the lower section in or near the lower inner zone.

The mother of the children placed her parents in a lower left-hand corner of the drawing. She reported that her connections to her family were never very good and that her parents had many problems while she was growing up and were now deceased. The mother indicated that her marriage had produced five children and that the father of the children was not a responsible man. She had married when she was very young to get away from her parents. Her ex-husband was physically and emotionally abusive and his current whereabouts was unknown. The mother guessed that he probably was deceased but she could not verify it. The mother shared that both she and her husband would drink alcohol on a regular basis and it made it difficult for them to provide a good life for their children. At this point the mother's three older sons who are now adults also had problems with alcohol and drugs and were not as connected to the family. The mother currently did not know where they were and had not seen them in many months. The mother included a symbol outside the family symbol but connected to the family drawing for the social worker that manages the family situation and makes decisions regarding foster care. The mother reported that the social worker is an important part of our family at this time. Other family members did not include the social worker.

Table 9.2 Step four, placement of others: zone and region, Example 9.A

Mother: red	M boyfriend: black	Sister 1: orange	Sister 2:green
Outside: Mother 7:00 Father 7:00 Children's father off 7:00 corner Son1 6:00 Son3 partial 7:00 Son2 partial 6:00 Foster mother 1:00, Foster father 1:00 Foster son1 2:00 Foster son2 2:00 Social worker 11:00 off to corner	Outside: Mother, Father 12:00 Foster mother 1:00 Foster father 1:00 Foster son1, Foster son2 2:00 Brother3, Brother2, Brother1 between 5:00 and 6:00	Outside: Foster mother, Foster father between 12:00–1:00 Foster son1, Foster son2 2:00 Brother1, Brother2, Brother3, partial 4:00	Outside: Foster mother, Foster father 1:00 Foster son1, Foster son2 2:00 Brother1, Brother2, Brother3 4:00
Outer: Brother3 partial 7:00 Brother2 partial 6:00	Outer:	Outer: Brother1, Brother2, Brother3 partial 4:00	Outer:
middle	middle	middle	middle
inner	inner	inner	inner

The mother's boyfriend also placed some symbols for his parents which indicated that he held them in high regard but that he was not close to them while growing up. Both of his parents were currently deceased. He also shared that his childhood home life was difficult. His symbols indicated that he saw things the ways his partner saw them as far as his partner's children and her experience of the foster family.

Both sisters shared similar experiences of the significant others in the family life space. The foster parents were experienced by both girls as outside the family symbol in a powerful position. The drawing suggests that they are not as emotionally close to the foster parents as they are to their mother. Both see their brothers in lower positions in the drawing. They do not know the brothers very well as all three brothers left home when the girls were very young. Foster care workers do not encourage contact due to the current lifestyle of the brothers.

Step Five: Environmental Symbols (Not Illustrated)

The mother placed symbols for recovery and her employment in positive locations close to the heart of family in the inner zone. The family placed symbols for the institution of foster care in the upper half of the family symbol and showed that it was in the 12:00 region indicating a significant placement of power over the family.

Step Six: Stress Symbols (Not Illustrated)

The mother placed significant symbols for stress connected to recovery and to a symbol that represented getting things right in her life. These symbols were relatively large and placed in the inner zone near the center of the family symbol. The sisters placed large symbols for stress related to losing their connection to their mother and getting out of foster care. These symbols were placed in the 12:00 region in the outer zone.

Using the FLSD With Case Example 9.A

The foster care worker used this drawing to process the situation within the family. The worker was able to see and hear that the two sisters were not interested in having parental rights terminated. The family lives in a state where the legal system considers the thoughts and desires of children in the process of terminating parental rights. The social worker was interested in learning about the familial connection of the girls and their mother through the FLSD. The girls were able to illustrate their sense of connection to their family of origin and their loyalties to a mother who has not always been able to effectively be responsible in providing adequate parenting. While in the assessment process, the mother expressed a strong desire to regain her parental rights and to live in a way that would be appropriate for her family. Using the information obtained from interactively exploring current dynamics with this family, the social worker decided to develop a plan for returning the children to their mother versus pursuing the termination of parental rights. Even though the foster parents had expressed a strong desire to adopt the two girls, the social worker decided to create another plan to help the family reunite. The treatment plan involved the mother following certain conditions that reinforced positive and responsible, safe long-term parenting.

Psychiatric Settings

Working with psychiatric patients can be a challenging and difficult process. Treatment orientations and processes that enhance the capacity of the people with severe mental illness to engage with the treatment provider will have the most success (Dixon, Holoshitz, & Nossel, 2016). The FLSD has the potential to engage patients with severe mental illness. Psychiatric patients present unique situations and need to be considered and treated with a client specific focus. Past therapeutic approaches to psychosis treatment included psychotherapy prior to the development of antipsychotic medications in the 1960s (Lauriello, Bustillo, & Keith, 2000). Even with the advance of the use of medication with psychotic patients some sort of supportive psychotherapy that takes into account the full needs of medical, social, and psychological interventions appears to be beneficial and useful in treating psychiatric populations (Gentile & Niemann, 2006).

Processing the psychiatric patients' situation with the FLSD will facilitate the important focus of the biopsychosocial process in client engagement. The FLSD's focus on identifying family members, environmental elements and issues related to stress cover all the areas of the biopsychosocial concerns. Psychiatric patients experience a hands-on tool that provides a nontraditional format for obtaining information. Previously developed defense mechanisms have the possibility of being diverted in the course of visually representing the patient's situation through the course of the drawing. Patients can let down their guards and create some representations that relate to their own life and situation. The interactive task process facilitates therapeutic alliance previously defined as an important element of patient's successful treatment outcome (Fluckiger, Del Re, Wampold, & Symonds, 2012). Interacting over the symbols placed in the FLSD create the situation where the person is able to express their specific personal experience. A good experienced facilitator of the FLSD will interact with the patient in a responsive and connecting manner. If the FLSD is conducted in an interactive process, the psychiatric client will feel heard and seen facilitating the alliance and successful treatment outcome.

The FLSD can be conducted with individuals to discover information about family history and also a way to identify the practical situation and potential need of the psychiatric client. Learning more about practical needs can be another way to enhance the engagement process of the psychiatric client (Dixon et al., 2016). The FLSD becomes a person-centered tool that can facilitate learning about the current strengths and needs of the patient. Taking time to interact with clients in the task of completing the FLSD will have advantages of sitting down with the patient with a clip board or the potentially boring process, for the client, of just answering questions off an intake form. The patient and the therapist or facilitator will interact and respond to each other thereby possibly creating a felt sense of connection.

The FLSD can be used to find out more information about the systemic elements of the psychiatric patient's family. The potential for placing previously unspoken information through the process of the drawing can help therapists develop curiosity about previously unknown and unexplored experiences in the patient's life. The visual representations can facilitate the creation of questions no one would have considered asking. Through the process of asking questions about the symbolic placements, the therapist facilitator can pursue new avenues of information with great potential for aiding the therapeutic process. The following example demonstrates the advantage of sharing information for a family where one member was currently undergoing treatment in a psychiatric facility. The FLSD allows for reinforcement of the individuation in families where the standard might be that all family members have the same experience of relationship. In this next example, sharing the individual perspective can be seen as having a dramatic affect.

Psychiatric Facility: Case Example 9.B

This case example presents a Caucasian male client aged 26 who is currently being treated in a psychiatric facility. He has experienced several hospitalizations related to dangerous violent outbursts in his home environment. Most of the violent outbursts in the past were directed at his father. Despite medication treatment he continued violent outbursts even in the hospital and sometimes required isolation to protect himself and others from the outbursts. His long-term treatment involved being seen individually by a psychiatrist who offered medication and supportive counseling support. As an adjunct to his individual treatment the psychiatrist decided to add a family evaluation session utilizing the FLSD process. The mother of this adult son joined the process. The father of the adult son had been deceased for about three years.

Step Three: Placement of Self

Key to Symbols

Mother

M: mother
H: husband
B1: oldest brother
B2: middle sibling
Dr.: staff psychiatrist
MM: mother's mother
MF: mother's father
GMGM: great maternal grandmother

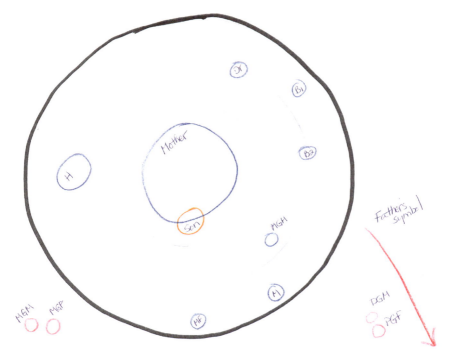

Figure 9.3 Steps three and four: placement of self and significant others, Example 9.B

Adult Son

M: mother
F: father
DR: staff psychiatrist
PGF: paternal grandfather
MGM: maternal grandmother
MGF: maternal grandfather
PGM: paternal grandmother

The mother started the placements and placed herself in the center of the inner zone as a very large symbol. As she drew her symbol she stated that she is in this location because she is holding the family together. Her adult son followed her and placed his symbol for self also in the inner zone at the 6:00 position. He placed his symbol partly overlapping in his mother's symbol. We have found that when adult people place symbols in another family member's symbol it is a strong possibility that the person has a lack of differentiation. It is not always limited to psychiatric patients but it is a symbol commonly seen in that population. Inner zone placements indicate a strong sense of family connection. Both of the family members completing this drawing see themselves in the inner zone and have a strong sense of connection to each other.

Step Four: Placement of Significant Others

The next phase of symbols placements involves Step four where family members place symbols for significant others. The mother placed her husband parents and a grandparent and siblings. Not all of these symbols on in the illustration. In addition, she identifies a great grandmother who lived with her in childhood. The adult son placed his father and his grandparents. Both the adult son and his mother placed the psychiatrist in the family drawing.

When the mother placed the symbol for her deceased husband she indicated that her husband was an "angel" and that he was a wonderful husband and father to their son. The placement

Table 9.3 Step three, placement of self: zone, region, and size, Example 9.B

Mother	Placement of self: Extra-large symbol inner zone center of zone
Adult son	Placement of self: Inner zone 6:00 average size

Table 9.4 Step four, significant others: zone and region, Example 9.B

Mother: blue	Adult son: orange
Outside: no symbols	Outside: Father across the room 5:00 direction PGF PGM 5:00, MGM MGF7:00
Outer: mother's father 6:00, mother's mother 5:00 Husband partially outer 9:00 Brother1 2:00 Brother2 partially 3:00, DR partial 1:00	Outer: no symbols
Middle: MGM 5:00, brother2 partial 3:00 Husband-9:00 Dr-1:00	Middle: DR 10:00 edge of zone
Inner: Self center	Inner: self 6:00

of the husband in the outer zone is a strong suggestion that the relationship between them was not as "wonderful" as she was indicating. The drawing suggests distance from all extended family members. She places her parents in a low position and these placements suggest poor or strained relationships. Of course, it is very important to offer that observation to verify if the client denies or supports the hypotheses. At the time of conducting the drawing the mother was not questioned about the possibility of distant relationships with her family of origin even though the drawing has some evidence of negative outer zone, lower placed connections.

The adult son placed his symbols for his family members outside the family symbol. When placing symbols outside the symbol it is usually an indication of very poor connections and relationships. Positioning symbols outside the 5:00 and 7:00 regions is a possible indication of low regard and emotional disconnection. When it was time for the adult son to place a symbol for his father on the drawing, he hesitated and walked away from the drawing over to another corner of the room 30–40 feet away from the drawing and stated that his father belongs here. The position was in a down position from the 5:00 region of the drawing. The adult son indicated that his father did not belong on the chart. When the adult son made this representation and statements about his father's placement the mother protested and became agitated. The mother immediately expressed surprised and told her son he was "wrong" and that he must be making the placement because he was "sick." She adamantly reminded her son that he and his father were really close and that his father was really a good man. As a result of his mother's outbursts and comments the adult son did not make any more symbolic placements and silently returned to his seat without challenging his mother. Normally this would be a good time for the therapist facilitator to remind family members that everybody has their own way of seeing things.

Step Four: Distance of Symbols

In this drawing the mother had her closest symbol to the doctor at 2.4 and her most distant relationship measure to her father at 5.5. The adult son in this drawing had his closet connection to his mother and his most distant connection to his father at an infinity measure mark away from his symbol.

Steps Five and Six: Environmental and Stress Symbols

The mother and adult son placed other symbols in the drawing related to the hospital. The adult son saw the hospital partially in the outer zone and partially outside the family at the 9:00 region. The mother placed the hospital symbol in the 12:00 position outer and middle zones of the symbols.

Step Eight: Communication Lines

The process of completing the communication lines in this drawing added a very important dimension to this family evaluation. Usually, the person will draw a line indicating good, so-so, or poor from their own symbols to others symbols on the drawing board. Sometimes this can be accomplished by the therapist or facilitator who will draw the symbols on another sheet of paper or make shortened notations; mother and her adult son drew their own symbols.

The mother drew good communication lines to her husband, son, and the doctor. She also drew good communication lines to her two of her brothers. She drew poor communication lines to her parents and so-so communication lines to maternal grandmother. She explained that her parents were distant and hardly ever home. She spent more time with her maternal grandmother during the time she was growing up.

When the adult son took his turn to draw communication lines he placed a good communication line to his doctor and a so-so communication line to his mother. He drew a line from his own symbol toward the direction of symbol for his father that he had previously placed across the room. The adult son became very emotional and dramatically started placing multiple hash marks on the communication line indicating poor communication. His mother challenged him but this time the therapist restrained her and the adult son was encouraged to sit in his chair. As the adult son, was in essence given permission to have his own experience, he was able to defend his position by explaining that he had some very painful experiences with his father. After completing these communication lines, the adult son was able to share information about being sexually molested by his father's friends. When the adult son was a young child, the father would take him to a local bar and offer him over to his friends for sexual exploitation. The adult son experienced the father as enjoying this event and was furious with his father for not protecting him. The adult son's mother initially protested these negative remarks about her husband but stopped speaking as she observed her son's emotional reaction. The symbolic representation of expressing a negative connection to his father, allowed the adult son a freeing experience to actually share new information about his childhood. Representing sexual abusers in a distant position from their own symbol in FLSD has been noted in past FLSD research (Barker, Barker, Dawson, & Knisely, 1997).

This revelation about being sexually abused was new information to both the Mother and the psychiatrist. The doctor had worked with the adult son for many years but had not heard anything about these types of experiences. After completing the FLSD the psychiatrist proceeded with a different approach to treatment for the adult son working with the after effects of being sexually traumatized. The new focus in treatment effort helped the adult son to make improved progress that facilitated leaving the hospital and interrupted the patterns that paved the path to repeated hospitalizations.

Completing the FLSD does not always lead to dramatic revelations and insights into unspoken family secrets. Even so we have seen the process be the vehicle for revealing information that is new to the people creating the drawing on many occasions. Geddes and Medway (1977) identified the process an experiential and cognitive blend that lowers defenses and allows people to express concerns and ideas in an indirect and nonthreatening way. In the case of this previous example, the presence of the supportive doctor and the FLSD process that facilitated his individuation in the room with the mother was a catalyst for safely sharing a painful experience. The process was specific to him and his own experiences. The adult son was able to show his unique experiences visually by his separate symbolic placements made with his own specific color. Having the therapist's attention and his own colored marker in a combined family session is a simple step toward creating a safe place for individuation. It also facilitated a step away from the possible enmeshment of adult son and mother that enabled the adult son to share the painful memories of experiences with his father.

School Settings

According to the American School Counselor Association, school counselors are employed to help students with academic, career, and social and emotional development (American School Counselor Association, 2018). School counselors interact with students around all aspects of the student's life. This involvement includes working as a team of educational and mental health professionals along with family members and parents.

School social workers and counselors have been able to use the process of the FLSD with students they are counseling in the school system. Individual students can complete a drawing to share information about not only how the student identifies family members but also to share information about environmental factors and stress issues in the ongoing aspects of the student's everyday life. The FLSD can identify types of social support and can be a means for investigating potential areas of concern. Lack of social support can be an indication of potential health risks and can be measured through simple applications of the FLSD (Blake & Bertuso, 1988). School counselors can take advantage of the FLSD to investigate the ecological environment of the student exploring direct and indirect messages in the symbolic placements.

Sometimes schools are able to invite the students' family into the school to complete a family assessment. These family meetings help to identify areas of concern that will facilitate the student in moving toward an effective role as a student in the educational system. Students can identify areas of environmental activities in the process of step five. They are also able to symbolically represent stresses and concerns through step six of the drawing process. Past FLSDs with students have seen the drawing help families recognize anxieties in the student concerning being over involved in activities and pressures related to learning disabilities. The visual representations helped families to see the load on the student and make effective changes in the student's environment. Other symbolic representations allowed for the symbolic identification of bullies in the neighborhood and school environment. The process can provide clues as to the severity of all the elements affecting student life. Exploring the symbolic placement as well as examining the size of the symbol placed in the drawing have sometimes helped identify potential risks for suicidal ideation and behavior. The combination of the visual medium as well as supportive verbal interactions facilitates the various learning styles of both students and parents.

Sometimes specialized services are offered in the school system for students with special needs. The following case example provides a demonstration of how the FLSD process facilitated a special needs student in obtaining vital family support. This example demonstrates the unique opportunities available in obtaining information in a nonverbal manner.

School Settings: Case Example 9.C

The next case presentation includes a middle-class African American family that includes two heterosexual parents and three children. The family was referred for counseling due to concerns about the youngest son, age 9, acting out in school. The child was referred for individual counseling but the therapist suggested a family session to evaluate the family situation. The youngest son was born deaf and was the only child in his class experiencing deafness. The child had learned American Sign Language (ASL) in a specialty school when he was very young and he had some support with ASL interpreters in the classroom. No one in the youngest son's family was able to sign effectively and as a result this child was often alone and isolated. The FLSD assessment included an interpreter for ASL.

Step Three: Placement of Family Members

Key

F: father, light blue
M: mother, red
D: daughter, age 16, dark blue
S1: son1, age 14, orange
S2: son2, age 9, green

Step Four: Placement of Significant Others (Not Illustrated)

Other significant family members included in the family drawing were grandparents and a family pet. Grandparents were placed in higher clock regions but located in the outer zone. The family pet was placed in the inner zone but in a lower region of 6:00 and 7:00.

Step Five: Environmental Factors (Not Illustrated)

The family members placed symbols for work and school and placed the symbols close to their own symbols.

Table 9.5 Step three: zone, region, distance, and size, Example 9.C

Person	Zone and region	Distance	Size
Husband: light blue	Outer zone: near middle between 4:00–5:00	13 cm Mother 4.2 cm Daughter 6 cm Son1 14.2 cm Son 2	similar
Mother: red	Outer zone: near middle at 9:00	13 cm Father 7.8 cm Daughter 8.2 cm Son1 11.5 cm Son2	similar
Daughter: dark blue	Half inner half middle 6:00	4.2 cm Father 7.8 cm Mother 0.4 cm Son1 9 cm Son2	similar
Son1: orange	Middle zone: 6:00	6 cm Father 8.2 cm Mother 0.4 cm Daughter 7.6 cm Son2	similar
Son2: green	Outside symbol: 7:00	14.2 cm Father 11.5 cm Mother 9 cm Daughter 7.6 cm Son1	similar

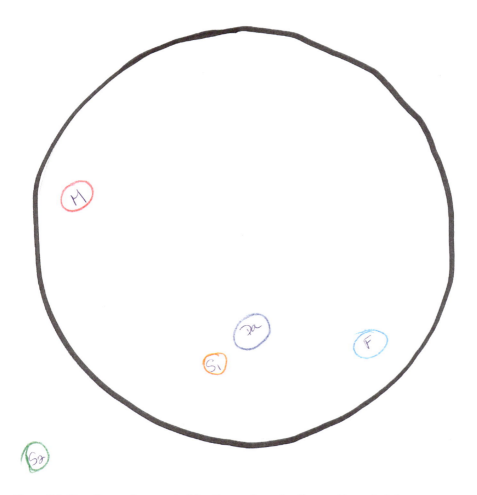

Figure 9.4 Step three, placement of family members: family case, Example 9.C

STEP SIX: STRESS SYMBOLS (NOT ILLUSTRATED)

The children placed stress symbols for school, and the parent's work, Son 2 placed symbols near each family member. Both parents placed stress symbols near their work and also placed average sized symbols in the inner zone explaining the symbol represented stress with life.

STEP EIGHT: COMMUNICATION LINES (NOT ILLUSTRATED)

The most telling demonstration in this family is when Son 2 was unable to draw any lines other than poor communication to his family members. Most of the other family members represented lines that ranged from so-so to poor. The two oldest siblings reflected good lines to each other.

Using the FLSD With Case Example 9.C

After completing the FLSD, family members were asked to comment on their experience in developing the FLSD. Family members expressed surprise when they were able to view the drawing and realize how isolated they were placed from each other. The people in the family were able to express for the first time how they noticed that they lacked a sense of connection. One family member stated "we all coexist in the same household but we don't feel like a family." Other family members expressed similar feelings and said they wanted more in terms of family relationships.

They talked about how Son 2 must feel about being so isolated and lonely because of his deafness. The value in having the entire family participate in the creation of a FLSD helped family members realize how isolated and alone Son 2 must feel. They were sensitive to Son 2's deafness but had not realized that their inability to communicate with Son 2 impacted so heavily on him. Son 2 informed his family about his experience by placing himself outside the FLSD isolating himself as if he were not a part of the family. Son 2's symbol is away from other family members. The position of a symbol outside the drawing in a low position usually indicates low self-worth and low self-esteem. When Son 2 was questioned through the signing interpreter, he confirmed that he had low self-esteem feelings about himself and his relationship to other family members.

After the family had an opportunity to comment on what each person observed and learned from participating in developing the FLSD, the therapist asked family members what the reason was for them coming to the therapy session. The father responded with the comment, "I thought we were coming here because of Son 2's problems at school. After this exercise, I realized that the problems are much broader than that one issue. It seems like all of us have issues that affect each one of us in the family." The therapist reviewed some of those issues. Son 2 placed himself outside the family symbol and expressed a sense of rejection and isolation. He stated that he did not feel like he was part of the family. This is an issue that all family members wanted to be aware of and address. The Interpreter suggested an ASL sign language class, that family members could attend so that they could learn to sign and communicate with Son 2. Family members agreed to attend classes in order to learn to sign. They were all concerned that Son 2 did not feel like he was included in the family.

Isolation in this family seems to be a pattern. Mother and father have a great distance between them which indicates marital conflict and avoidance. All of the other family members seem to occupy isolated positions on the FLSD. The majority of the space considered the heart of the family is empty of people and It is occupied by stressors. The mother and father expressed a desire to improve their marital relationship and wanted to become more active in their leadership roles.

Son 2's isolation issues with the family and his difficulties at school were clearly identified in this family session. All family members expressed concern that they could visually see that Son 2 felt excluded from the family and they wanted to help him feel part of the family. All agreed that they would enroll in the ASL class and learn to sign so they could better communicate with John. All family members agreed to continue family therapy not just for Son 2 but for the entire family.

Treating the Mental Health Needs of Deaf Culture

The FLSD is uniquely positioned to help address the needs of a nonverbal population by providing a visual expressive modality for communication. It is understood from the World Health Organization (2018) that 466 million people worldwide have disabling hearing loss and 34 million are children. Providing mental health services to deaf individuals requires a cultural competency in the areas of deaf culture and a sensitivity to provide special communication provisions for the deaf. Using certified interpreters is important if the therapist is not ASL proficient. The advantage of the FLSD is that a deaf client is able to transmit nonverbal information through their own expression by placing symbols related to their felt sense of experience.

This case example family demonstrates the common issue that over 90% of significant others in a deaf person's life are unable to sign and provide a language model when that child is born into the family (Williams & Abeles, 2004). Using the FLSD adds a significant tool to allow for deaf individuals to express symbolically and directly in a visual language. Interpreters can help to explore the meaning of the symbolic representation when the therapist is not proficient in ASL. The use of the FLSD can help to minimize some of the inherent and potentially unethical problems that arise when working with interpreters because the client is placing their own symbols and communicating their own message. People working with the deaf culture have been aware of the need for tools that help to measure psychological issues in a language compatible with the deaf culture (Boness, 2016). While the FLSD process with this family still required an interpreter, the therapist and family were able to discover a visual image that helped bring about significant change in this family. The FLSD has great potential in providing an expressive tool for nonverbal populations.

The visual image of seeing the family member outside the family symbol had a dramatic effect on the family. While they were aware of communication difficulties within the family they did not effectively translate that experience to a desire to learn communication techniques that would facilitate better connections. Viewing the information presented in the FLSD helped the family to see disconnected relationships and a visually demonstrated picture of low self-esteem for all family members. Learning a new language and beginning to embrace aspects of deaf culture helped the family feel better about themselves. The facilitating therapist also decided to learn ASL to assist with future work with this family.

Summary: The FLSD in Human Services Settings

The process of the FLSD has been used in various in human services settings and programs. In addition to social services, psychiatric facilities, and schools, the FLSD has been used for helping people with substance abuse issues, hospice, and families in need of intensive home based services to name a few. The FLSD provides a low keyed expressive technique that enables the therapist or counselor to join the clients in any service program by going beyond traditional question and answer forms to interacting with clients in a systemic way. Clients can symbolically represent concerns that become the focus of treatment. An example might be in the area of substance abuse issues. The issues can be graphically represented in the FLSD process and the visual can be utilized to investigate the experience of the client. The visual representations can direct the development of treatment plans.

All age groups and populations can use this process. Even when people have different physical abilities the drawing can adapted to whatever physical situation the client may have in allowing them to complete the process. We have used the FLSD with elderly populations and children as young as age 4 and have always brought the drawing to the level of whatever the person needed as an adjustment. The biggest limitation for using this process might be with people unable to see the visual aspects of the drawing board, though we have used this process with people who previously had sight and can direct placements via the clock image. As a general rule this process would be difficult for people who have visual limitations but not totally impossible as people without sight can verbally represent images and other geometric symbols even though the person has never been able to use sight to know the symbol.

One of our strongest premises is that the FLSD has great potential in helping clients and therapists or counselors create a connecting experience where they can mutually symbolically, visualize the family situation through the creation of the FLSD. After completing the drawing clients will have a sense that the counselor knows about their background and has information pertaining to the life stresses that bring them to counseling. If the client includes many family members each person has been afforded individual attention and has had a platform for individual expression of systemic issues facing the individual and family members. Clients who have had previous counseling experiences without first using the FLSD have reported that the FLSD process was a fun way to share information and that they were able to share more in that one session when it took many weeks in other types of therapy.

In reviewing essential elements of family assessment by various authors we see the FLSD covering all of the important elements of family assessment. Thomlison (2016, p. 30) informs that the assessment process includes gathering, analyzing, and synthesizing relevant data about the family. The relevant data should include information about stressors, and strengths and resources. The FLSD process is not just an information gathering process but includes a recognition and examination of dynamic forces and unspoken elements depicted in the assessment process. Nichols and Tafuri (2013) suggest that assessment is learning about the families point of view and also challenging them to consider other possibilities.

Finally, and most importantly the process of the FLSD facilitates the process of engaging the client by providing a vehicle that enables the client to achieve a sense of being connected to the therapist by expressing spoken and unspoken messages through the interactive process of reviewing family members, environmental issues and life stressors. This sense of connection is identified as joining (Patterson et al., 2009). The development of an effective alliance and connection appears to be one of the most critical factors in the process of future treatment (Sundet, 2011; Fluckiger et al., 2012; Wampold, 2015). The interactive process of the FLSD allows the therapist and client to co-create a client specific reference that standardized measure have difficulty in facilitating (Lavee, 2006).

These important elements of family assessment can be transferred to any setting that seeks to provide counseling support in human services. This chapter has provided some brief examples of the potential use of the FLSD in specialized settings. It would be difficult to discover a counseling setting that could not take advantage of using the FLSD process with clients. The visual representation of the holistic picture of the family is a great opportunity to experience the world of the client and to begin the helping process.

REFERENCES

American School Counselor Association. (2018). Retrieved from www.schoolcounselor.org/parents-public

Barker, S. B., Barker, R. T., Dawson, K. S., & Knisely, J. S. (1997). The use of the family life space diagram in establishing interconnectedness: A preliminary study of sexual abuse survivors, their significant others and pets. *Individual Psychology*, 53(1), 433–450

Blake, R. L., & Bertuso, D. D. (1988). The life space drawing as a measure of social relationships. *Family Medicine*, 20(4), 295–294.

Boness, C. L. (2016). Treatment of deaf clients: Ethical considerations for professional psychology. *Ethics Behavior*, 26(7), 562–585.

Child Welfare Information Gateway. (2017). *Foster care statistics 2016*. Washington, DC: US Department of Health and Human Services, Children's Bureau. Retrieved from www.childwelfare.gov/pubs/factsheets/foster/

Deacon, S. A., & Piercy, F. P. (2001). Qualitative methods in family evaluation: Creative assessment techniques. *The American Journal of Family Therapy*, 29, 355–373.

Dixon, L. B., Holoshitz, Y., & Nossel, I. (2016). Treatment engagement of individuals experiencing mental illness: Review and update. *World Psychiatry*, 15(1), 13–20.

Fluckiger, C., Del Re, A., Wampold, B., & Symonds, D. (2012). How central is the alliance in psychotherapy? A multilevel longitudinal meta analysis. *Journal of Counseling Psychology*, 59(1), 10–17. https://doi.org/10.1037/a0025749

Geddes, M., & Medway, J. (1977). The symbolic drawing of the family life space. *Family Process*, 16, 219–228.

Gennari, M., Tamanza, G., & Accordini, M. (2015). Family life space: Emerging couple and family relations. *Procedia Social and Behavioral Science*, 165, 94–102.

Gentile, J. P., & Niemann, P. (2006). Supportive psychotherapy for a patient with psychosis. *Psychiatry (Edgemont)*, 3(1), 56–61.

Lauriello, J., Bustillo, J., & Keith, S. J. (2000). Commentary: Can intensive psychosocial treatments make a difference in a time of atypical antipsychotics and managed care? *Schizophrenia Bulletin*, 26(1), 141–144.

Lavee, Y., & Avisar, Y. (2006). Use of standardized instruments in couple therapy: The role of attitudes and professional factors. *Journal of Marital and Family Therapy*, 32(2), 233–244.

Lesser, R. P. (1982). Stress and illness in the family: A linear versus family life space perspective. In D. Mostwin (Ed.), *Ecological therapy: The family life space approach*. Baltimore, MD: Loyola College.

Mostwin, D. (1980a). *Social dimension of family treatment*. Washington, DC: National Association of Social Workers.

Mostwin, D. (1980b). Life space approach to the study and treatment of a family. In D. Mostwin (Ed.), *Life space approach to the study and treatment of a family*. Washington, DC: The Catholic University of America.

Nichols, M., & Tafuri, S. (2013). Techniques of structural family assessment: A qualitative analysis of how experts promote a systemic perspective. *Family Process*, 52(2). https://doi.org/10.1111/famp.12025

Patterson, J., Edwards, T. M., Chamow, L., & Grauf-Grounds, C. (2009). *Essential skills in family therapy: From first interview to termination*. New York, NY: Guilford Press.

Sundet, R. (2011). Collaboration: Family and therapist's perspectives of helpful therapy. *Journal of Marital and Family Therapy*, 37, 236–249.

Thomlison, B. (2016). *Family assessment handbook: An introduction and practical guide to family assessment* (4th ed.). Boston, MA: Cengage.

Wampold, B. (2015). How important are the common factors in psychotherapy? An update. *World Psychiatry*, 14, 270–277.

Williams, C. R., & Abeles, N. (2004). Issues and implications of deaf culture in therapy. *Professional Psychology Research and Practice*, 35(6), 643–648.

World Health Organization. (2018). Retrieved from www.who.int/news-room/fact-sheets/detail/deafness-and-hearing-loss

CHAPTER TEN
Family Life Space Drawing and Research: Past, Present, and Future

Research and the FLSD

As in many areas of counseling the process and uses of the FLSD developed from an informal research stance that derived from the scientific process of learning through the direct experience of being in the world (Heppner, Kivlighan, & Wampold, 1992, p. 5). Mostwin and her graduate student teams employed the practice of the FLSD and collected many observations about the placements, size of symbols, and patterns noticed over the years of practice. Mostwin shares some of those observations about the meanings of symbolic placements in her writings, and we have discussed them in previous chapters (1980, p. 62). Models of family therapy practices in the 1970s were not as concerned with adherence to methods based in research as much as practitioners are in recent times. As a result, the observations were not systematically recorded with a research protocol mindset to allow us the advantage of having a structured research process to support the observations and assumptions about the FLSD tool. Mental health practitioners did not always connect research based practice to their choice of interventions and needed to be encouraged to follow research based designs in treatment and counseling tool choices (Heppner et al., 1992, p. 28). The authors support the value of research to investigate the validity and best uses of the FLSD and are hopeful for the potential revelations that future research will bring.

Despite the lack of a structured process to record observations, some of Mostwin's students engaged in research to investigate the effectiveness of the short-term family therapy they were utilizing in the internship counseling center. This chapter will review some of the student research and review some of the research related to using the FLSD as a research tool. In addition, this chapter will include some information about pilot studies currently in process that attempt to compare visual representations with standardized measurements.

Early Research of Short-Term Multidimensional Family Intervention (STMFI) and the Family Life Space Drawing (FLSD)

Mostwin's major focus in developing the FLSD was to provide a systemic and holistic means of engaging and meeting families in the early stages of a short-term dynamic directive therapy with predelinquent youth (Mostwin, 1982a). The initial research efforts were concerned about the effects of the STMFI therapeutic interventions. These efforts evaluated positive outcomes in terms of the youth avoiding criminal behavior and parents adopting more traditional roles as heads of the household. The earliest research focused on evaluating whether or not the families improved their functioning.

A descriptive article by Geddes and Medway (1977) encouraged the use of FLSD beyond the STMFI model. This article described the FLSD process using symbol placements for individuals and social institutions involved with the family life space. The process did not include psychological or stress symbols at that time. The article also suggested the use of communication lines to help define and clarify the clients experience as they completed the drawing. These authors suggested that the FLSD could serve as a diagnostic source that provides:

1. Information about family structure
2. A tool that would gauge intrafamilial congruence
3. A research device measuring change in family structure.

The article also provided some case examples and suggestions for using the FLSD process.

The master thesis research of Allman and Madigan (1974) focused on observing outcomes of six families who participated in the STMFI treatment while participating as clients of the Family Studies Center of the Catholic University of America. Dr. Mostwin was the supervisor and teacher for student interns at the center. Sometimes nonstudent professionals participated on these teams of therapist working with families. The research evaluated the goals of the therapy, which were to help families improve communication patterns, change role perceptions, and achieve completion of assigned tasks and goals defined in the process of the therapy.

This study originally used the FLSD as a research tool to evaluate the pre- and post-changes in communication within the family. The research would evaluate changes in communication lines pre- and post-treatment. The student researchers ended up rejecting the FLSD tool as measurement device because they judged that the definitions of the symbolic terms had not been standardized. The student researchers were also concerned that the use of the process to help diagnose the family was also a challenge to the reliability of the measure.

The final results of the Allman and Madigan study showed that most of the families achieved some of their treatment goals. One family achieved 100% of their goals while the lowest score for achievement was 22% of goals achieved. The clients reported a mean result of moderately being happy with the treatment. Two of the families showed a significant score or adopting improved congruency in familial roles questionnaire scores used in the process of the study.

Continuing the investigation of the FLSD as a potential research device, Dailey (1980a) designed a study for his master's thesis that evaluated first and last session drawings of 27 families treated at the university's Family Studies Center. Dailey focused his research on measuring the location of the family members in treatment and looking for a sense of closeness and cohesion as represented after treatment by his measures. Dailey took a compass and obtained diametric measures of all of the family member's symbols within the drawing and hypothesized that the diametric measures would be smaller or tighter after completing treatment (Dailey, 1980b). He also thought that the center of the circles would rise and family members would be placed higher in the family drawing after completing treatment. The results of this study demonstrated that the families did have closer symbols in the final drawing versus the first drawing at a 0.001 significance level ($t = 5.383$, 26 df). In one example clients moved away from the edges of the drawing and close to each other near the center. In almost every example, family drawing configurations changed after completing treatment. The study results did not support the second assumption that the family members would change positions to a higher position in the final family drawing. Dailey concludes his research findings as offering that the STMFI treatment model helps to improve family closeness.

Mostwin (1982b) published a case study of 13 families involved in a community project attempting to design interventions that would help predelinquent youth. Mostwin (1982b) used the FLSD as a way of illustrating the families' situation at the start of treatment and at the end of treatment. To evaluate the effectiveness of the treatment Mostwin had 13 judges who viewed presentations of the cases from the treatment team and rated the families on a rating scale from 0 to 93. The scale ratings indicated deterioration at 0 and major improvement at 93. None of the families in the case study group rated as, situation greatly deteriorated. The study results showed that 38.4% of the study families improved, 38.4% improved greatly, and one family solved its problems through the course of treatment. Mostwin did not evaluate the FLSD diametrically to determine closeness in the way that Dailey had previously evaluated his study.

In our recent post-study examination of the eight example drawings in the 1982 case study, it appears that the eight illustrations of her first and final sessions shows most of the families measuring closer when examining the diametric measures suggested by Dailey (1980a). We compared the two diametric measurements of family symbols before and after treatment using a t test calculation and showed a statistical significance of change. The value of t is -7.631539, and the value of p is 0.000123. The value is significant at $p \leq 0.05$. Statistical examination of the Wilcoxon Signed Rank Test also showed a critical value of W for $N = 8$ at $p < 0.05$ is 3, therefore the result is significant at $p \leq 0.05$. These results reveal that family configurations do change before and after treatment of the STMFI model. The actual meaning and emerging properties of those changes are not measured.

THE FLSD AS A RESEARCH DEVICE

The FLSD was used as a research tool to assist with medical interventions by defining the number of good social connections and comparing that number to health risk potentials (Blake & Bertuso, 1988). A nurse practitioner used the FLSD symbols for people and institutions along with communication lines. The study participants were 93 women who had previously participated in a stress management prevention program. The stress management program included a FLSD in the first session. The study randomly selected the 93 women and categorized social connections and communication lines related to those communication lines. The study found that the women with more poor connections and relationships had higher morbidity than those women who had positive relationships and good connections with their social network. The authors stated that higher morbidity was noted in those without a spouse or significant other as well as those with a poor relationship with a spouse or significant other. This study result was in line with other studies that noted that the positive quality of partner connections affect the women's health positively according to the authors. The authors also noted that the use of the FLSD helped the stress management program to identify areas that they could address in developing new areas of the stress management program. The authors of this article reflect that the use of this tool has been a preliminary investigation and that the tool required additional research to help support its use.

Barker and Barker (1988) began a series of studies that utilized the FLSD as a measure of emotional closeness. All of the studies included a focus on the importance of pets to social connections (Barker & Barker, 1988; Barker, Barker, Dawson, & Knisely, 1997). One study also expanded the study of dog owners and attempted to study the construct validity of the FLSD (Barker & Barker, 1990).

The FLSD served as a research tool to measure emotional closeness to human relationships as well as pets. The authors measured distance between the symbols in the FLSD drawing, assuming that projective measures in art therapy indicated distance and closeness as previously demonstrated by art therapist Okoniewski (1984). The study measured distances between the symbol for self and the symbol for pets or other significant family members. The study evaluated 122 people and showed that the respondents drew themselves as close to their pets as they did their family members (Barker & Barker, 1988). The study is suggesting that pet bonds may be as strong as family bonds. One of the useful aspects of this study is to begin the measurement of distance between the symbols as a possible indication of closeness.

The measurement of symbol placements continued in the subsequent article by Barker and Barker (1990) with the addition of providing adjectives that would describe the relationship between the symbol for self and pets and significant family members. The researchers provided additional reports concerning information obtained in the 1988 study that was attempting to serve as a validity tester for the study results. After completing the FLSD and placing only symbols for self and significant others the participants were asked to draw lines to their symbols and to place descriptive words that would express their sense of the relationship. The researchers rated the 219 descriptive words obtained in the study as emotionally close or not emotionally close. The data measurements of the actual distance of the symbols of the person drawing the FLSD to symbols for significant others were combined with descriptive words identified as words for closeness or words for disconnection. The results indicated that study participants who placed symbols close to themselves also used descriptive words that supported the concept of emotional closeness. Symbols for family members or pets who were drawn farther away from their own symbol were also described in words that represented distant or not close relationships. This is an important study to support the construct validity of the FLSD as a measure of emotional closeness. The researchers support the use of the FLSD as a quick and easy technique that can serve as a springboard for exploration of various family relationships (Barker & Barker, 1990).

In a creative application of using the FLSD for research, Barker et al. (1997) used the FLSD as a graphic representation of the childhood past of 40 sexual abuse survivors. The study participants ranged in age from 20 to 50. The participants included men and women from both Caucasian and African American backgrounds, as well as one person who self-identified as an "other." The participants were clients of four different therapists who completed the drawings with their clients. The study participants were asked to place symbols for the significant people and pets from their childhood. After placing the symbols, the study participants were given a scaled number choice that corresponded to a word for abusive or supportive. The scaled number choices were from 1 to 7. The researchers again measured the distance between the symbol for self and symbols for significant others. They used a mixed-models repeated-measure analysis of variance. The study also noted qualitative aspects of the placements of responders looking for patterns and locations placed in the drawings.

The study results indicated that symbols of greater distances from the symbol for self were also noted as symbols described as abusive. The more abusive the relationship was described, the more distance the symbol would be from the symbol for self. The researchers described commonly observed patterns in drawings that suggested that survivors will place supportive symbols near them and the abusers far away from their own cluster of supportive symbols. This study also indicated that pets are more likely to be symbolically placed as supportive. The authors suggest that using the symbolic placements of significant others is an effective way to provide some distance when talking or reflecting on difficult topics such as childhood sexual abuse. The article notes that the symbolic placements can serve as a beginning place for asking questions about the symbols and experiences with those people and pets placed in the drawings (Barker et al., 1997).

The research offered by the Barkers illustrates the potential usefulness of measuring family connections and evaluating those family members as close or not close. Using the measurement of distance between symbols would provide an opportunity to review the closeness measurement before treatment and after treatment. This type of consideration would be useful in working with couples. The suggestion that symbols close to the symbol for self-indicate closeness to the symbol for self is a good starting point for conversations with clients.

More recently, the FLSD has been utilized as a research device by Italian researchers Gennari, Tamanza, and Accordini (2014). The researchers have used the FLSD to explore couple and family relationships among migrant populations coming to live in Italy from Morocco, the Philippines, and Pakistan. The researchers used the FLSD in three iterations that to represented past family configurations, present relational patterns and future family configurations. The 66 participants were asked to draw three different FLSD that included communication lines for how they were in the past, are now in the present, and how they wanted the family to be in the future. Their research was able to see how the families might be currently functioning and the possibilities for future transformations in the family. The study used Mostwin's definition of positive positioning by looking for representations of inner zone positions in the FLSD as strong indicators of effective couple functioning (1980). The study also explored the presence or absence of social relationships both in the past home country and in the current host country. The results of the study defined four categories of immigrant couples. The researchers identified category one couples as being capable of making positive adjustment as evidenced by strong connections to each other and positive connections to the past home country and the new host country. The researchers developed a second category of couples who had good connections in their homeland but no meaningful connections in the host country. Couples in this category were also not positioned in the center of the drawing but have a vision of positive connections for the future. The third category of couples were those who do not have placement in the center of the drawing and reveal good social connections in the country of origin but have rigid visions for the future. The fourth category of couples show a greater distance between the couple symbols and symbols for self. The symbols are not connected and represent their social connections in the homeland and host country as separate from each other. The future drawings of this fourth category of couples show no difference in the past and future drawing leaving the researchers to assume that the couples have limited vision for improving future possibilities.

The researchers used the symbolic representations as a way to understand the potential problems facing these migrating couples. The researchers suggest that the FLSD can be a process that helps to identify the stage the couple or family might be dealing with in the process of migration adjustments. The researchers also reflect that the FLSD was very useful in working with the problems related to language differences. Symbolically placing symbols allowed couples to depict information that they might not have direct words to express.

Other Uses of the FLSD in Research

Coogan (1982) demonstrates that the FLSD has the potential to help adolescent boys reveal their life situation on a holistic level and identify symbolically social relationships that have a strong influence on them. Wirsching (1976) reports that his agency was able to utilize the STMFI model to reduce teen referrals to courts from 57% to 10%. This report credits the use of the FLSD as a means of facilitating diagnosis, providing clues as to unspoken issues and a measurement of movement within the family. Banning, Ferraro, Lothamer, and Yeakel (1980) reveal that the FLSD can be a useful tool in exploring cultural and ethnic issues for families facilitating therapist sensitivity and cultural competencies.

Researching Expressive Graphic Techniques

Graphic and expressive techniques have been utilized in marital and family therapy for assessment and interventions since the early interventions were first utilized (Nichols & Tarfuti, 2013; Thomlison, 2016). While the use of standardized measures of psychological scales and paper scored tests have been used in assessing individuals for mental health counseling, family, and marital counselors have been reluctant to take on the use of standardized measures (Lavee & Avisar, 2006). They suggest that standardized measurements do not meet the needs of therapists in clinical practice. Deacon and Piercy (2001) also expressed this concern that quantitative measurements did not completely evaluate or reveal the holistic nature of families. Deacon and Piercy (2001, p. 358) offer that qualitative assessment methods that include graphic techniques and tools can encourage the following advantages to assessment.

1. Active self-reflection
2. Assessment and therapy directly complement each other
3. Qualitative assessment can be chosen to "fit" therapist's theory
4. Qualitative assessment is shared assessment
5. Qualitative assessment empowers
6. Qualitative assessment increase the family commitment to the assessment and therapy process
7. Qualitative assessment supports family communication and understanding
8. Qualitative assessment provides a holistic contextually rich sense of the family
9. Qualitative assessment is flexible for use with diverse families
10. Qualitative assessment uses the family's own personal constructs.

This list delineating the value of qualitative assessment measures illustrates the potential contributions of the FLSD. The qualitative components of this process allow it to be client specific, holistically, flexible, and co-constructed by therapist and client with unique client information. While it may be difficult to develop normative standards for the FLSD in the way that standardized assessment tools offer, the process does provide a clinical tool that helps to initiate the therapy process.

Graphic instruments are difficult to research due to the unique and nonnormative aspects of the various drawings (Creswell, 2003). Despite the difficulty in developing standardized reference points, some researchers have found value in using graphic instruments such as genograms and ecomaps due to the positive clinical outcomes that arrive as a result of completing the graphic process with the clients (Watts & Shrader, 1998; Ray, 2005; Rempel, Neufeld, & Kushner, 2007). These studies suggest that benefits of using the graphic instrument involved co-constructing and collaborating with the client as well as discovery of information about supportive networks that the visual tool facilitated.

Future Research

We recognize that the FLSD has some research potential that has not been realized. The potential of examining the underlying aspects of the meaning of symbols in the drawing might have some value in applying a normative standard for the symbolic placements. Mostwin and her early teams of therapists and students began to observe some patterns that have held up for them over the years in understanding clients and families.

Mostwin developed the FLSD with inspiration from field theory with the recognition that person plus environment equals life space. Lewin (2013) developed this concept further by envisioning a geometric process where human behavior and psychology could be mathematically categorized. He developed formulas that examined behaviors through measurements of opposing forces, measurements of valences, determining structure of force fields, overlapping force fields, force and potency of a situations (Lewin, 2013). Those of us who have utilized the FLSD have never investigated those mathematical formulas to investigate the potential information from the spatial illustrations in the FLSD. Such a process could be developed by those who understand the complicated mathematical applications of Lewin. Other researchers have examined the graphic results of art therapy and the FLSD could use coding grids much in the way that Gennari and Tamanza attempted with conjoint family drawings (2013).

Research could compare the FLSD with standardized measures much in the way that Calix (2004) did when attempting to show construct validity of the ecomap. Users of the FLSD could continue the before and after therapy intervention methods of comparing drawings at the start and end of therapy employed in past research, this comparison could be valuable in discovering if families were able to develop some structural change as observed by Dailey (1980a).

FLSD Pilot Studies

As practitioner researchers, the authors have begun some small-scale pilot studies with couples seeking relationship counseling to compared our FLSD with some standardized surveys to see how they support information from each other. Couples completing the surveys agreed to have this information revealed with identifying information absent. We plan to continue these studies that will compare the FLSD with various other measurements. The authors also plan to develop a study program that will use the FLSD as measurement of before and after treatment.

These studies are examples of our attempts to apply a research process to the FLSD. We recognize that the studies only provide preliminary information and present the raw data as a demonstration of what a research comparison might look like in terms of data collections.

The FLSD examples are copies of actual drawings of the pilot study participants who agreed to participate in the standardized measure comparisons. The drawing includes faint images of the zones to allow the reader to see the placement zones for understanding client placements. In actual drawing the zones are not apparent to the client and the circle is often a roughly drawn circle.

Pilot Study One: Family Assessment Measure (FAM-III) and the FLSD

Three couples, a total of six people, who were seeking marriage counseling participated in the study. The study compares the drawings in terms of measured spatial connections to spouse, parents, and significant family members with the quantitative scores of a self-report instrument the Family Assessment Measure (FAM-III). This study utilized scores from a shortened version of the FAM called the brief FAM-III. The shortened version of all scales showed a Cronbach's alpha score of over 0.80, indicating a good internal consistency (Skinner, Steinhauer, & Sant-Barbara, 1995). The FAM-III measure provides a numeric score concerning family functioning strengths and weaknesses. The measure was designed to provide information concerning the process model of family functioning that integrates various approaches to family therapy and research, but has been used to measure other types of family interventions (Skinner et al., 1995). The FAM-III measures (1) General Scale, focuses on family as a system; (2) Dyadic Relationships, relationship between specific pairs; and (3) Self-Rating Scale, relates to individual's perception of functioning in the family. The measure was found to have significant scores for determining discriminant validity, construct validity, and clinical validity (Skinner, Steinhauer, & Sitarenios, 2000). The interpretation of the FAM-III reports that scores of 50 indicate average level of family functioning. Scores higher than 50 indicate more than average family difficulties. Scores over 60 indicate greater difficulties with family functioning and score below 50 indicate healthier family functioning with scores below 35 described as excellent.

In this study, we are comparing scores related to relationship, self-esteem and family functioning with information we would obtain from FLSD and see how it compares. The information from the FLSD will be presented in terms of position and size of person on the drawing, along with measurements of distance between significant family members.

FAM-III and the FLSD: Couple Case Example 10.A

This Caucasian couple in their early fifties was married 1 year ago and sought marriage counseling at the time of the surveys to deal with marital issues related to his ex-spouse and teenage child. Both members of the couple were employed in highly educated positions and both had achieved significant accomplishments in their chosen profession.

Steps Three and Four: Placement of Self and Significant Others

Key to Symbols

Male: blue   Female: green
M: self   F: self
MD: daughter, age 14   FS: female's son, age 24

Mo: mother
F: father
FW: father's wife
B1: brother 1
B2: brother 2
BW: brother's wife
EW: ex-wife
B3: brother 3

M: mother
F: father
B: brother
Ex-H: son's father
BW: brother's wife
S: sister
SH: sister's husband
N & N: nieces and nephews

The partner's drawing indicates that they are closest to their children at 2.5 cm for him and 1.2 cm for her. They are most distance from ex-spouses at a distance of 7.7 cm for him and 6.5 cm for her. Placing of symbols at close range can indicate a strong sense of connection and family bond (Barker & Barker, 1990). The distance they have from each other is 7.5 cm and is among the most distant measures in the family drawing. The female places her symbols for significant family members near her in close range but outside the family symbol. The placement at 7:00 might indicate some low self-esteem and a position of low power and significance in this family grouping. Placing symbols for significant others might indicate that she has not integrated her extended family into this family system.

FAM-III Scores: Couple Case Example 10.A

The scores of the FAM III are interpreted according to the following scale:

65 or above Problematic

56–64 Increasing problems

45–55 Average

36–44 Increasing strengths

35 and below Excellent

Table 10.1 Steps three and four, placement of self, significant others: region, zone, size, and distance, Example 10.A

Male partner: blue	Female partner: green
Location of self and size: 10:00 region middle zone, partial inner and partial outer. Large symbols for self and others	Location of self and size: 7:00 region outer zone and middle zone. Large symbol for self, smaller for others
Significant others: Father and Fa Wife 11:00 outside Brother 3 Outside 2:00	Significant others: Female's son 7:00 outside
Mother 12:00 outer zone	Mother 7:00 region outside
Brothers1, 2 12:00 outside	Father 7:00 outside
Brother4 and his wife 1:00 outside	Siblings 7:00 outside
Sister outside and outer zone	Ex-husband 7:00 outside
Ex-wife outside 4:00	Nieces/nephews 7:00 outside
Daughter middle and outer zone 4:00	
Distance: Father 2.5 cm	Distance: Son 1.2 cm
Mother 3.5 cm	Father 2.5 cm, Ex-Husband 6.5 cm
Brother1 6.5 cm, Brother2 5.3 cm, Brother4 3.5 cm, Brother's wife 3.7 cm	Mother 3 cm, Nieces/nephews 3.2 cm
Spouse 7.5 cm, Pet 2.5 cm	Brother 4.5 cm, Brother's wife 3.9 cm
	Sister 2.5 cm, Sister's husband 2.3 cm

FAMILY LIFE SPACE DRAWING AND RESEARCH

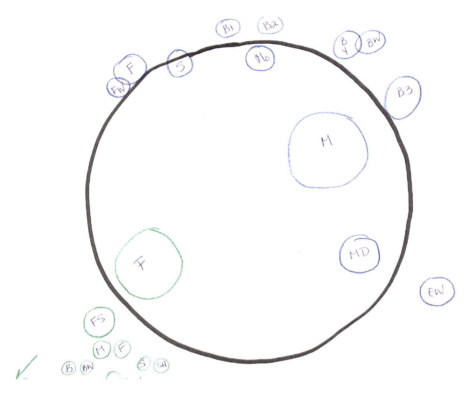

Figure 10.1 Steps three and four: placement of self and significant others, Example 10.A

Table 10.2 FAM-III scores, Example 10.A

Couple 1 Female	Couple 1 Male
Dyadic 50	Dyadic 49
Self 70	Self 48
General 60	General 46

This couple's score indicate that they are operating at different level of family functioning in the surveys areas. He scores in the low average range in all his scales with the dyadic scores the closest to showing problematic functioning. The wife's scores indicate problematic functioning in all scale scores.

The visual representation of the FLSD would be congruent with the sense of self score as revealed by the wife's placement in the lower half of the family symbol in the outer zone of the family symbol. Placing symbols in this lower position usually indicates a low sense of power or function in the family. Her position away from the family center in the symbol as well as placing her significant family members is an indication of her general disconnection from the family. The survey scores indicate problems in this area. Of greatest concern is the distance between the partners away from the inner zone.

FAM-III AND THE FLSD: COUPLE CASE EXAMPLE 10.B

The next drawing is from a Caucasian couple in their mid-thirties seeking marriage counseling due to stress about parenting differences in regard to their two children. Both of the spouses work outside the home. They indicated stresses about the children and personal issues, and the marriage.

STEPS THREE AND FOUR: PLACEMENT OF SELF AND SIGNIFICANT OTHERS

Key to Symbols

Female

F: Female spouse
FM: Female's mother
FF: Female's father
FD: Female's daughter
FS: female's son

Male

M: Male spouse
MM: Male's mother
MD: Male's father
MDA: Male's daughter
MS: Male's son

The female is close to all of her symbols but is closest to her son with the drawing showing an overlap of symbols. The farthest symbols are for her father and her daughter both located either in the inner zone or quite close to it. The overlapping symbols typically indicate an undifferentiated closeness indicating that she is potentially over involved with the son. She places herself in the center inner zone indicating a place of emotional connection and responsibility. The most distant symbols in this drawing are between the male and female partners who place themselves 5.5 cm apart. Sometimes partners will draw each other closer if given a chance to draw symbols for each other. It is standard in this process to ask the partners to refrain from drawing symbols for each other.

Table 10.3 Steps three and four, placement of self, significant others: region, zone, size, and distance, Example 10.B

Female: green	Male: blue
Location of F Self and Size: Center of the inner zone, large symbol	Location of M Self and Size: outside and outer zone large symbol 7:00
Significant others: symbols smaller than self	Significant others: symbols smaller than self
Female's mother: inner middle zone 11:00	Mother: middle outer 7:00
Female's father: inner middle zone 12:00	Father: middle 7:00
Female's son: inner 9:00	Son: middle 9:00
Female's daughter: inner 6:00–7:00	Daughter: inner 3:00
Distance	Distance
Mother 0.3 cm, daughter 1 cm	Mother 0.5 cm, son 5.5 cm
Father 1 cm, son overlap	Father 0.2 cm, daughter 7.2 cm

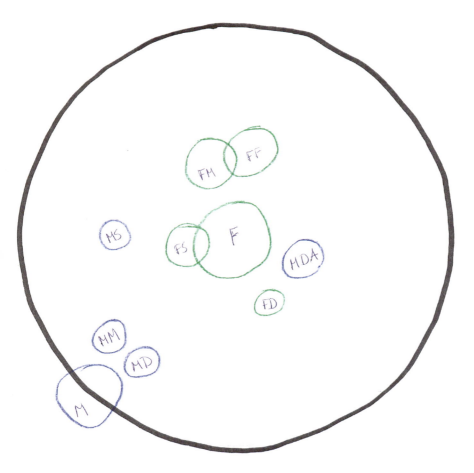

Figure 10.2 Steps three and four: placement of self and significant others, Example 10.B

The male in this drawing also had symbols for his parents close to him with very little space between his parent's symbols. He placed the symbols for children at the most distance from him but placed them close to the emotional center of the drawing near the symbol for his wife. The male in this drawing placed all of his symbols above him making him the lowest symbol in this drawing. His placement for self, typically represents a lower position of power and sense of self. Even so his large sized symbol represents a good sense of self. He may think he is in the doghouse of the relationship.

FAM-III Scores: Couple Case Example 10.B

The scores for this couple indicate increasing problems for the dyadic relationship and problematic functioning for the other two scales (see scale on page 344). Both partners scored in similar ranges to each other-possibly indicating that they see the family situation in relatively the same way. Scores of 60 and above indicate difficulties with family functioning (Skinner et al., 1995)

Table 10.4 FAM-III scores, Example 10.B

Chapter10 Couple 2 Female	Chapter 10 Couple 2 Male
Dyadic 62	Dyadic 62
Self 66	Self 68
General 72	General 68

The FLSD indicates that the couple has some major disconnects from each other in that they have a large distance between their symbols. The lower 7:00 position, partially outside the family symbol, that the husband draws for himself represents an area of concern for family functioning. He places himself away from the family center and his wife and children. The male is close to his own family of origin but significantly distant (when compared to his parents) to symbols for his wife and children. He has his greatest distance between himself and his children's symbols and the symbol of his wife. Another potential concern is the female's overlapping symbol of the son. Overlapping symbols sometimes indicate an over involvement or over identification with that person. The FLSD would agree with the FAM-III assessment.

FAM-III and the FLSD: Couple Case Example 10.C

The last couple reviewed with the FAM-III, is a Caucasian couple where one is 60 and the other one is 51. The couple was seeking marital counseling to cope with stress. This is a second marriage for both of them and neither of them have children. This couple owns two successful businesses and has a hobby concerning specialty hunting dogs. The completed drawing for this couple was full of large symbols for environmental elements (step five) affecting the couple. The stressors (step six) mostly concerned issues of disorganization and being overwhelmed. (Steps five and six are not illustrated here.)

Steps Three and Four: Placement of Self and Significant Others

Key to Symbols

Female	Male
F: female self	M: male self
FD: female's father	MD: male's father
FM: female's mother	MM: male's mother

The couple has some very large symbols for self and slightly smaller symbols for others. The others in this situation are their parents who have all passed away. The symbols for the couple are very close together in or near the inner zone. Both of the partners take up a lot of space in this drawing as do their symbols for their deceased parents. The closest symbols in the drawing are for each other indicating a sense of connection for each other. Her farthest symbol is for her mother at 2 cm away from her symbol. These distances would be considered close. The male's most distant symbol is for his father who is across the family symbol from

Table 10.5 Steps three and four, placement of self, significant others: region, zone, size, and distance, Example 10.C

Female: green	Male: purple
Location of F Self and Size: A large symbol in the center of inner zone	Location of M Self and Size: large symbol inner, middle, and outer zone 3:00
Significant others size: Mother middle zone 12:00, large but smaller than her symbol Father middle zone 11:00, large but smaller than her symbol	Significant others: large symbols Mother outer middle zone 11:00–10:00 Father outer middle zone 9:00–10:00
Distance: Partner 0.8 cm Mother 2 cm Father 1 cm	Distance: Partner 0.8 cm Mother 8 cm Father 8.5 cm

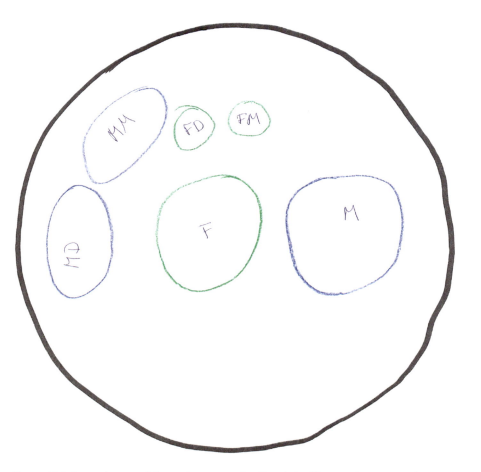

Figure 10.3 Steps three and four: placement of self and significant others, Example 10.C

Table 10.6 FAM-III scores, Example 10.C

Female couple 3	Male couple 3
Dyadic 50	Dyadic 46
Self 50	Self 48
General 52	General 38

his own symbol. The male places his father and mother in positions of respect but in this drawing it does show some disconnect.

FAM-III Scores : Couple Case Example 10.C

The scores for this couple indicate average levels of functioning on all the scales. Scores higher than 50 indicate increasing problematic situations and the smaller the score the better the situation concerning functioning (see page 184 for full scale).

The symbols in the FLSD support the FAM-III average functioning level scores as we see the couple close together in the emotional center. Both are located in the upper regions of the family symbol indicating a positive sense of self. His FAM-III scores indicated that he is functioning at an average level of family functioning. He supported this concept by indicating that he is happy as long as his wife is happy. At this point, life events and involvements were the inspiration to seek counseling interventions. The FLSD provided more information to the clinical assessment than this survey measure by showing us that the couple is close but that there may be some problems due to his location toward the outside zone of the family symbol.

Summary of FAM-III Results and the FLSD

The initial results of comparing the FLSD symbol representation in terms of spatial position, size, and symbol distance from partners suggest that the two measures can match each other and have some comparable results when evaluating average functioning or disconnects.
This early study is suggestive but interesting to us as we evaluate the information from both sources. Comparing a numeric measure with a graphic evaluation is a difficult comparison but not so different in that we can discuss both types of evaluations. The authors recognize the limitations of such evaluations but we are interested in comparing the results. Calix (2004) developed a numeric score for eco-maps in order to compare the graphic measure with other standardized surveys. A similar process could be developed for the FLSD but for now we are left with discussing the visual results with a standardized measure.

Pilot Study Two: FLSD Compared to Experiences in Close Relationship Survey (ECR-R)

This pilot study compared the FLSD with a standardized measure for attachment connections. The study used an attachment survey based on an original survey by Hazan and Shaver (1987) used to inform on attachment experiences in romantic relationships. This revised edition is the Experience in Close Relationships-R (ECR-R), a 36-item measure that provides two subscales related to anxiety and avoidance reporting on their experience with their partner's availability or avoidance (Fraley, Waller, & Brennan, 2000). The internal consistency reliability for this scale tends to be 0.90 or higher (Sibley & Liu, 2004, p. 973).

People with higher levels of anxiety in relationship are likely to score higher on this scale, with a score of 7 rating as highly anxious. Anxious individuals are concerned with rejection and tend to worry about being abandoned. People who have a high score in the avoidant scale are not as likely to seek intimacy and desire independence. Higher scores on either scale point to higher levels of anxiety and avoidance. The greater the likelihood of being anxiously or avoidantly attached the more difficult it is to manage stressful emotions.

This review compares FLSD from three couples, six people with their scores for the ECR-R surveys. The FLSD information is reported only in terms of placement of self and significant others. The couples were seeking relationship counseling and agreed to participate in the study comparison by completing the surveys. The information is presented with limited identifying information.

FLSD and the ECR-R: Couple Case Example 10.D

This Caucasian heterosexual couple (male aged 33 and female aged 31) sought relationship counseling to better understand each other. They had been married in the last year and were feeling disconnected. Her parents were divorced in her childhood and her primary caretaker was her mother. He grew up with both parents and had a sibling.

Steps Three and Four: Placement of Self and Significant Others

Key to Symbols

M: male
MM: male's mother
MD: male's father
FR: friend (5) S: sibling
F: female
FM: female's mother
FD: female's father
FR: friend

This couple created a drawing with both of them on opposite sides of the drawing. They are placed in high positions possibly indicating a higher sense of self. Each of them has drawn their significant others close to them. They appear to be out of the family center possibly indicating that they have not formed a family identity between themselves. The symbols with the greatest distance in this drawing are between the couples themselves. Each of the partners in this drawing symbolize themselves in a separate section of the family. The male partner has created a circle of people around him consisting of friends. Both of them have symbols for people around them in an almost barrier like fashion.

ECR-R Scores, Anxiety, and Avoidance: Couple Case Example 10.D

The two subscales for anxiety and avoidance show the partners scoring opposite in relation to the subscales. The male had higher scores for avoidance than his female partner. She scored higher on the anxiety measure than the male partner.

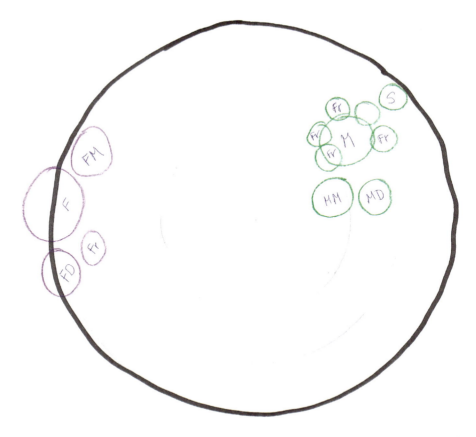

Figure 10.4 Steps three and four: placement of self and significant others, Example 10.D

Table 10.7 Steps three and four, placement of self, significant others: zone, size, region, and distance, Example 10.D

Male: green	Female: purple
Location of self and size: He is in middle zone between 1:00 and 2:00 region; average size symbol	Location of self and size: Outside and outer zone at 9:00; average size symbol
Significant others: Size smaller than self Mother: inner and middle 3:00 Father: middle zone 3:00 Sibling: outer zone 2:00 Friends: smaller middle zone some partial outer 2:00	Significant others: Size similar to self Fr is smaller Mother: Outer zone 9:00–10:00 Father: Outside and outer zone between 8:00–9:00 Friend: Outer zone and middle zone between 8:00–9:00
Distance: from partner 11.5 cm Mother 0.8 cm Friend overlap symbols Father 1 cm Sibling 0.5 cm	Distance: Mother: zero distance touching Father 1 cm Friend 1 cm

Table 10.8 ECR-R scores for anxiety and avoidance, Example 10.D

Female	Anxiety 3.4	Avoidance 2.5
Male	Anxiety 2.4	Avoidance 3.6

According to this measure both of the partners score in a relatively securely attached score range. The concept of secure attachment indicates that partners in this range are comfortable being close to their partners and do not have many concerns with rejection.

FLSD and ECR-R Comparisons: Couple Case Example 10.D

The ECR-R scores show some congruencies with some of the FLSD indications. The couples are located in the high regions of the FLSD and located in positive placements. The size of symbols in the FLSD indicate a positive sense of self as do the secure attachment scores on the ECR-R. The interesting aspect of the ECR-R scores provides some insight as to the opposite placements of the partners. The male partner scores higher in avoidance and the female higher in anxiety. These opposite adaptations may contribute to the evidence of distance in the FLSD. The opposite adaptation strength may be a factor in the couples not "understanding" each other and the reasons they were seeking counseling in the first place.

FLSD and ECR-R: Case Example 10.E

The next comparison of the two measures reviews the drawing of a Caucasian heterosexual couple in their fifties who are in their second marriage. Each member of the couple had children prior to his marriage and also had a child together. The youngest child is still in high school. Both members of the couple have deceased parents. The male partner has been treated for alcoholism but is not currently abstaining from alcohol. They are seeking couples therapy due to issues with effective communication and intimacy

Steps Three and Four: Placement of Self and Significant Others

The couple completed this drawing symbolically placing themselves in lower positions in regions reflecting potential low sense of self and personal power. The mostly adult children are placed in the inner zone or closer to it by both partners in this couple.

Key to Symbols

M: Male partner
MM: male's mother
MD: male's father
MS: male's son

F: female
FF: female's father
FM: female's mother
FMD: female's daughter

Table 10.9 Steps three and four, placement of self, significant others: zone, region, size, and distance, Example 10.E

Male: blue	Female: green
Location of self: outer middle zone 7:00 region	Location of self: middle/inner 4:00
Size: largest symbol	Size: largest symbol
Significant others: size parents larger than other symbols	Significant others: size slightly smaller
Father: outer zone 6:00	Mother: inner zone 3:00
Mother: inner 6:00	Father: inner zone 3:00
M Son and partner: middle zone 8:00	MF daughter: middle zone 3:00
Daughter and partner: middle/inner zone 7:00	Female son: center inner zone 3:00
Male's female daughter: inner zone 6:00	Male daughter: inner zone 3:00
Female's son: 6:00	Male son: inner zone 3:00
Distance: partner 7 cm, MDA 2 cm	Distance:
Father 2 cm, female son 3.6 cm	Mother 1.2 cm, male son 3.6 cm
Mother 2.6 cm, MF daughter 2 cm	Father 0.8 cm, male daughter 5.6 cm
Male son 0.2 cm	MF daughter 1 cm

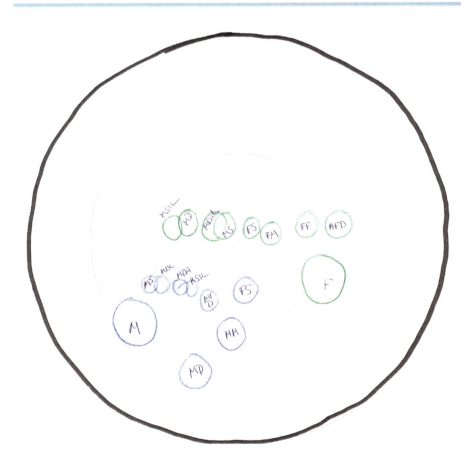

Figure 10.5 Steps three and four: placement of self and significant others, Example 10.E

Blank symbol: partner to child   MS: male's son
FMD: female's daughter   MD: male's daughter
FS: female's son
MFD: male's female daughter   Blank: spouses of stepchildren

The couple also has some grandchildren not included in this representation of the drawing. This drawing shows us that the inner zone includes the children for this couple representing the emotional connection and significance of these children to the family concept. Both of the partners see the children in a significant place. The couple has the greatest distance between themselves. Please note that if a partner was asked to draw their partner in the drawing there is a good chance that the drawing would include that symbol closer than the way it is currently represented. In this instance, it helps us to notice the distance and the low sense of self between the couple. Noticing these representations allows us to begin a treatment conversation. For research purposes, we see significant distance between the couple and a low sense of family position in each partner, with the Female partner having a slightly higher sense of family position self. She also has some connection with her symbol to the inner zone of the drawing representing emotional connection to the family center. Both partners have a sizable symbol which indicates a good sense of self but not in the role and relationship of this family group.

ECR-R Results: Couple Case Example 10.E

The ECR-R survey measures report on two subscales related to anxiety and avoidance. The scales indicate that a higher score indicates high avoidance or anxiety and low scores indicate low anxiety and avoidance. Sometimes these scores can be translated to measures of being insecurely attached in relationships.

This measure shows the female partner scoring in the securely attached zone and the male partner in the less securely attached zones of measurement. This indicates a difference in attachment styles.

FLSD and ECR-R Comparisons: Couple Case Example 10.E

The male partner symbolized himself in the lower half of the circle partially in the outer zone. This could be reflective of his subscale score with a higher range of anxiety and avoidance. The difference in attachment styles could also be reflective of the communication difficulties identified by the couple. The FLSD indicates some spatial difference in the couple with their relationship distance the greatest distance between all the symbols. Having a slight tendency to insecure attachment can create opportunities for not being able to rely on the partner in a time of emotional need (Johnson, 2013).

Table 10.10 ECR-R subscale scores, Example 10.E

Female	Anxiety 2.27	Avoidance 2.33
Male	Anxiety 4.6	Avoidance 4.0

FLSD AND ECR-R: COUPLE CASE EXAMPLE 10.F

Steps Three and Four: Placement of Self and Significant Others

This review of the FLSD and ECR-R measure of Couple 6 shows a Caucasian couple both in their thirties. They have been married for 4 years but have been in relationship for 6 years. Currently they have a 9-month-old son. They are having relationship issues and are seeking counseling to improve connections. Both have living parents who remained married to each other and who live in close proximity to the couple. This drawing includes symbols for each of the partners and their own representations of their son. The drawing includes some of the significant others such as parents and siblings and a pet.

Key to Symbols

M: male   F: female
MM: male's mother   FM: female's mother

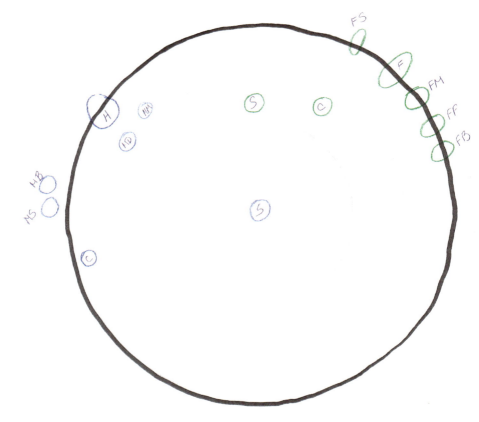

Figure 10.6 Steps three and four: placement of self and significant others, couple case, Example 10.F

MD: male's father   FF: female's father
S: son   S: son
MB: male's brother FS: female's sister
MS: male's sister   FB: female's brother
C: cat   C: cat

This drawing has the couple located in upper regions indicating a strong sense of self and regard in the highest regions of the drawing. They place themselves and symbols for significant others close to their own symbols. The exception is their 9-month-old son, who is placed in the center of the family drawing. His symbol is the most distant symbol for her placements. The male also places the symbol as one of the most distant of all his symbols. Both partners indicated the infant son is a strong reason for them working out relationship difficulties. Environmental and stress symbols were placed in this drawing mostly in the center of the drawing. She placed large symbols for her home and faith taking up most of the space in the family symbol. These symbols are not illustrated in the drawing example.

ECR-R Scores: Case Example 10.F

The two scores for anxiety and avoidance are indicated in the chart below. The higher scores for either scale indicate greater anxiety and avoidance related to attachment connections.

The measures on these scores reflect a potential for a negative view of the other and a slight tendency to a less secure attachment for both of the partners. They both indicate higher scores for anxiety versus avoidant behavior.

Table 10.11 Steps three and four, placement of self, significant others: zone, size, and distance, Example 10.F

Male: blue, size average	Female: green, size average
Location of self: outside and outer zone 11:00 and 10:00	Location of self: outside outer zone 1:00–2:00
Significant others:	Significant others:
Son: center of inner zone	Son: middle zone 12:00
Mother: outer zone-11:00	Mother: outer and outside 2:00
Father: outer zone 10:00	Father: outer and outside 2:00
Sister: outside 9:00	Sister: outer and outside 1:00
Brother-outside 9:00	Brother-outside and outer 2:00–3:00
Cat: 9:00–8:00	
Distance:	Distance
Wife 9 cm	Son 6 cm
Son 7.2 cm	Mother 0.6 cm
Mother: 1 cm	Father 1.7 cm
Father: 1.8 cm	Brother 3 cm
Brother 4.5 cm	Sister 1.5 cm
Sister 6 cm	Cat 2.6 cm
Cat 7.5 cm	

Table 10.12 ECR-R scores, Example 10.F

Female	Anxiety 4.5	Avoidance 4.0
Male	Anxiety 5.2	Avoidance 4.4

FLSD and ECR-R Comparisons: Case Example 10.F

The FLSD indicates a good sense of self but a great sense of disconnection from the partner. The higher scores in anxiety could be a good explanation for the distance between the couple. Both partners have trouble feeling securely attached to each other and this is reflected in the FLSD measure for distance. This couple have had difficulty forming a family identity as evidenced by symbolic placements in the outer and outside zones. The somewhat higher anxiety and avoidance scores could also reflective of lack of safety between the couple to allow for family formation.

Summary of Pilot Studies

These pilot studies reflect some of the inherent difficulty of researching graphic measures. All of the FLSD were client specific and there are many limitations in applying standardized interpretations to the drawings. Even standardized measures have limitations such as are reflected by Fraley et al. (2000) when they observe that the ECR-R is better at identifying insecure attachment than it is secure attachment. Applying interpretative meaning to FLSD also has some limitations in that the meaning applied by Mostwin (1980) and her students have not been systematically studied. The interpretations can only be suggestive.

In these pilot studies, we can see connections between the information learned from the studies but we also recognize that the connections can be born out of a desire to apply such a connection. In these few comparisons, we can see couples with secure attachments show distance between each other on the FLSD. It is possible that secure attachment does not necessarily prevent relationship difficulties. Or it could be that the secure attachment measure of the ECR-R is not adequately measuring the distress in those people that fall into the secure categories as mentioned by (Fraley et al., 2000).

It is possible that the standardized measures are not good measures to help research the component parts of the FLSD. All of the studies pertained to couples so the standardized measures related to relationship interactions. The FLSD has application in working with clients other than couples. It may be that the standardized measures need to be more connected to measuring factors in families. Even the FAM-III was designed to measure a process oriented family therapy intervention and the measure is related to that specific intervention. Both the FAM-III and the ECR-R are suggested as measures that need to be given to the client as a way to chart progress and changes in treatment. The FLSD has also been used in this type of fashion to examine therapy progress by Mostwin (1980) and others such as Dailey (1980a), Gennari et al. (2014).

Future Research

There is no question that the FLSD needs to continue its investigations of the actual meaning of its constructs. The big question concerns the most effective way to complete that investigation. The FLSD has been used as a way to measure change by evaluating differences in before and after treatment drawings. We are interested in learning more about the drawings ability to reflect family connections, and self-esteem. We would like to know if placements in certain zones truly reveal what we are currently assuming that it does. For example, does placing a symbol outside the family symbol truly indicate that the person does not feel like a part of the family? We would like to know more about our supposition that small or large symbols have significance as to the person placing the symbol's sense of self or the object or person placed in the drawing. We are also interested in exploring the concepts developed by Barker and Barker (1990) that placing symbols at a distance from your own symbol indicates a lack of closeness to that symbol or object. A challenge to that concept may be demonstrated in our example of Couple 10, where we see the mother of a baby place the child in the center of the drawing between her symbol and her husband's symbol when they as a couple are far apart. We know in this instance that she is close to her baby, but sees the baby placed in the emotional center. In combined family drawings, it is possible that positions in the emotional center mean something different than in individual drawings which Barker and Barker examined in their research. It is possible to question and explore differences individual drawing's unique manifestation compared to combined family drawings. It will be valuable and interesting for future research to reveal the potential of the FLSD to provide more definite information in regards to those concepts and interpretations related to it constructs.

Future researchers could develop mathematical formulations such as those developed by Lewin and to help inform about the meaning of distances and placements in the FLSD. In the future, it is possible that the structural configurations of families can lead to the development of categories after exploring a series of drawings for measurements of distances between family members. There are many future possibilities for exploring and attempting to standardized the meaning of the FLSD.

In the meantime, clinicians will have to take our suggestions for interpretations as suggestive and let the specific clients provide the basis for interpreting the results of the drawing. As always, the final meaning and interpretation of the drawing is left to the responses of the clients. If the clients find a way to experience the therapist as an interested, concerned human being willing to provide support and guidance along the way in the counseling relationship, then the outcome of the FLSD will be a successful event.

Summary

The Family Life Space Drawing has attempted some exploration about the value of its ability to assess and measure progress in family client interventions. In the past, FLSD measures were taken before and after family interventions. These early research efforts demonstrated that families did change positions in the drawing and that the symbols became closer after interventions. The graphic illustrations of the FLSD were also used to research social relationships and explore the possible connections of family relationships and social support in connection with sexual abuse. The FLSD has been used as a research device to measure family connections in the past and present and has been used with immigrant populations and patients in health service settings.

Despite the difficulties of researching a graphic personally expressive device, it is important to research the FLSD process and explore what the symbols might be conveying to therapists and clients.

REFERENCES

Allman, M. A., & Madigan, M. P. (1974). Presentation of some of the research findings from master thesis. In D. Mostwin (Ed.), *NCSSS seminar on social casework in the field of family treatment.* Washington, DC: The National School of Social Service.

Banning, F. M., Ferraro, F., Lothamer, J., & Yeakel, J. (1980). The meaning of cultural heritage: An exercise in sensitivity. In D. Mostwin (Ed.), *The life space approach to the study and treatment of a family.* Washington, DC: The Catholic University of America.

Barker, S. B., & Barker, R. T. (1988). The human canine bond: Closer than family ties? *Journal of Mental Health Counseling,* 10(1), 46–56.

Barker, S. B., & Barker, R. T. (1990). Investigation of the construct validity of the family life space diagram. *Journal of Mental Health Counseling,* 2(4), 506–514.

Barker, S. B., Barker, R. T., Dawson, K. S., & Knisely, J. S. (1997). The use of the family life space diagram in establishing inter-connectedness: A preliminary study of sexual abuse survivors, their significant others and pets. *Individual Psychology,* 53(4), 435–440.

Blake, R. L., & Bertuso, D. D. (1988). The life space drawing as a measure of social relationships. *Family Medicine,* 20, 295–297.

Calix, A. R. (2004). *Is the ecomap a valid and reliable social work tool to measure social support?* Master thesis. Baton Rouge, LA: Louisiana State University. Retrieved from https://digitalcommons.lsu.edu/gradschool_theses/3239

Coogan, J. L. (1982). The teenage view of life space. In D. Mostwin (Ed.), *Ecological therapy: The family life space approach.* Baltimore, MD: Loyola College.

Creswell, J. W. (2003). *Research design, qualitative, quantitative, and mixed methods approaches* (2nd ed.). Thousand Oaks, CA: Sage Publications.

Dailey, K. (1980a). *A preliminary evaluation of the family life space diagram: A life space approach.* Unpublished master thesis. Washington, DC: The Catholic University of America.

Dailey, K. (1980b). The use of the life space diagram in treatment. In D. Mostwin (Ed.), *Life space approach to the study and treatment of a family.* Washington, DC: The Catholic University of America.

Deacon, S. A., & Piercy, F. P. (2001). Qualitative methods in family evaluation: Creative assessment techniques. *American Journal of Family Therapy,* 29, 355–373.

Fraley, R. C., Waller, N. G., & Brennan, K. A. (2000). An item response theory analysis of self-report measures of adult attachment. *Journal of Personality and Social Psychology,* 78(2), 350–365.

Geddes, M., & Medway, J. (1977). The symbolic drawing of the family life space. *Family Process,* 16, 219–228.

Gennari, M., & Tamanza, G (2013) Conjoint family drawing; A technique for family clinical Assessment. *Procedia: Social and Behavioral Sciences,* 113, 91–10.

Gennari, M., Tamanza, G., & Accordini, M. (2014). Family Life Space (FLS): Emerging couple and family relations. *Procedia: Social and Behavioral Sciences,* 165, 94–102 https://doi.org/10.1016/j.sbspro.2014.12.609

Hazan, C., & Shaver, P. R. (1987). Romantic love conceptualized as an attachment process. *Journal of Personality and Social Psychology,* 52, 511–524.

Heppner, P. P., Kivlighan, D. M., & Wampold, B. (1992). *Research design in counseling.* Pacific Grove, CA: Brooks Cole.

Johnson, S. (2013). *Love sense.* New York, NY: Little, Brown, and Company.

Lavee, Y., & Avisar, Y. (2007). Use of standardized assessment instruments in couple therapy: The role of attitudes and professional factors. *Journal of Marital and Family Therapy,* 32(2), 233–244. doi.org/10.1111/j.1752-0606.2006.tb0102.x

Lewin, K. (2013). *The conceptual representation and the measurement of psychological forces.* Mansfield Centre, CT: Martino Publishing.

Mostwin, D. (1980). *Social dimension of family treatment.* Washington, DC: National Association of social Workers.

Mostwin, D. (1982a). Predelinquent youth and their families. In D. Mostwin (Ed.), *Ecological therapy: The life space approach.* Baltimore, MD: Loyola College.

Mostwin, D. (1982b). Life space of predelinquent youth and their families: An experimental community project with an ecological perspective. *International Journal of Family Psychiatry,* 3(3), 259–288.

Nichols, M., & Tafuri, S. (2013). Techniques of structural family assessment: A qualitative analysis of how experts promote a systemic perspective. *Family Process,* 52(2), 207–215. https://doi.org/10.1111/famp.12025

Okoniewski, L. (1984). A comparison of human-human and human-animal relationships. In R. K. Anderson, B. L. Hart, & L. A. Hart (Eds.), *Proceedings of the Minnesota-California Conferences on the human-animal bond* (pp. 251–260). Minneapolis, MN: Center to Study Human-Animal Relationships and Environments.

Ray, R. A. (2005). Ecomapping: An innovative research tool for nurses. *Journal of Advanced Nursing,* 50(5), 545–552. https://doi.org/10.111/j.1365-2648.2005.03434.x

Rempel, G. R., Neufeld, A., & Kushner, K. E. (2007). Interactive use of genograms and ecomaps in family caregiving research. *Journal of Family Nursing,* 13(4), 403–419. https://doi.org/10.1177/1074840707307917

Sibley, C. G., & Liu, J. H. (2004). Short-term temporal stability and factor structure of the revised experiences in close relationships (ECR-R) measure of adult attachment. *Personality and Individual Differences,* 36, 969–975.

Skinner, H. A., Steinhauer, P. D., & Santa-Barbara, J. (1995). *Family assessment measure: FAM III: Technical manual* (pp. 1–77). North Tonawanda, NY: Multi-Health Systems.

Skinner, H. A., Steinhauer, P. D., & Sitarenios, G. (2000). Family Assessment Measure (FAM) and process model of family functioning. *The Association for Family Therapy and Systemic Practice,* 22, 190–210.

Thomlison, B. (2016). *Family assessment handbook: An introduction and practical guide to family assessment* (4th ed.). Boston, MA: Cengage Learning.

Watts, C., & Shrader, E. (1998). How to do (or not to do) the genogram: A new research tool to document patterns of decision-making, conflict and vulnerability within households. *Health Policy and Planning* 13(4), 459–464.

Wirsching, W. (1976). *New dimensions in the juvenile service unit. The social dimensions of family treatment.* Washington, DC: The Catholic University of America.

Index

Note: Page numbers in italics indicate figures and in bold indicate tables on the corresponding pages.

Accordini, M. 178
Ackerman, N. 8–9
aging services, FLSD in 156–157
Allman, M. A. 175
American School Counselor Association 167
American Sign Language (ASL) 167–171
anxiety and Experiences in Close Relationship Survey (ECR-R) a 189–191
Anyal, A. 29
art therapy, family 35
Avisar, Y. 154
avoidance and Experiences in Close Relationship Survey (ECR-R) a 189–191

Banning, F. M. 179
Barker, R. T. 55, 155, 177–178
Barker, S. B. 55, 155, 177–178
Becvar, D. S. 34
Becvar, R. J. 34
Berrien, K. 30
Bertalanffy, L. von 29, 30
Bing, E. 35
blended families, FLSD with 125–140
Boszormenyi-Nagy, I. 8, 31
boundary zones 33
Bowen, M. 4, 13, 30
Bowenian therapy 4

Calix, A. R. 8, 180
Chamow, L. 14, 49, 153
Circumplex Model of Family Assessment 10, 16
Clark, R. 26, 44, 54; on greatest frustrations symbol 56

cognitive behavioral family therapy 10–11
Collins, W. A. 36
communication lines symbol 48, 48–49; in FLSD with couples 103–104; in FLSD with families 137–139; in foster care and termination of parental rights 165–166; in individual FLSD 85–86, 93; in psychiatric settings 165–166; in school settings 169–170
communication theory 34–35
control circle 51–52, *52*
Coogan, J. L. 179
counseling settings, FLSD in 153–157; deaf clients and 167–171; foster care and termination of parental rights 154–161; psychiatric 162–166; school 167–170; summary of 171–172
couples, FLSD with: communication lines in 103–104; environmental symbols in 100, **100**, *101*, 108–111, **109**, *109*, **110**, 119–121, **120**, *120*; Experiences in Close Relationship Survey (ECR-R) and (*see* Experiences in Close Relationship Survey (ECR-R)); Family Assessment Measure (FAM-III) and (*see* Family Assessment Measure (FAM-III) and FLSD); heterosexual, married, middle-class 104–114; introduction to 95; placement of self in 96, **97**, *97*, 104, **105**, *105*, 114–116, **115**, *115*; placement of significant others in 96–100, *98*, **99**, 106–108, **107**, *107*, 116, 116–119, **117**; research on 178; same-sex 95–104; stress symbols in 101–103, **102**,

102, 111–113, **112**, 112, 121–124, 122, **123**; summary of 124; unmarried parents 114–124
cultural dimensions of STMFI 23
cybernetic function of behavior 34

Dailey, K. 175, 176, 180, 196
Dattilio, F. M. 10
Davis, S. D. 4, 8–10, 12, 31
Dawson, K. S. 155
Deacon, S. A. 154, 179
deaf clients 167–171
Dicks, H. 8
distances and closeness of symbols 55, 165
Dyadic Adjustment Scale 10

Ecological Model of intervention 26–27
ecomaps 7–8, 9
Edwards, T. M. 14, 49, 153
emotional suppression 7
environmental symbols 47, **64**, 64, 64–66; in FLSD with couples 100, **100**, 101, 108–111, **109**, 109, **110**, 119–121, **120**, 120; in FLSD with families 131–134, 132, **132–133**, 145–148, 146, **147**; in foster care and termination of parental rights 161, 165; in individual FLSD 76, 76–77, **77**, 82–83, **83**, 83, 89–91, **90**, 90; in psychiatric settings 165; in school settings 168
Experiences in Close Relationship Survey (ECR-R) 188–189; heterosexual couple 189–191, 190, **190–191**, 194, 194–196, **195–196**; second marriage, heterosexual couple 191–193, **192**, 192, **193**
experiential model of family counseling 7–8
expressive therapy techniques 35

families, FLSD with: blended 125–140; communication lines in 137–139; environmental symbols in 131–134, 132, **132–133**, 145–148, 146, **147**; intact, with child having problems in school 140–152; introduction to 125; placement of self in 126–128, **127**, 127, 141, 141–142, **142**; placement of significant others in 128–131, **129**, **130**, 130, 142–145, 143, **144**; stress symbols in 134–137, 135, **135–136**, 148–151, 149, **150**; summary of 151–152

Family Adaptability and Cohesion Evaluation Scale (FACES) 10–11
family art therapy 35
family assessment 3–4; common components of 13–14; crucial qualities of effective 15; purpose and value of 14
Family Assessment Measure (FAM-III) and FLSD 181; marriage counseling due to stress and parenting issues case example **184**, 184–186, 185, **186**; marriage counseling due to stress in middle age couple 186–188, **187**, 187, **188**; middle-age couple case example 181–184, **182**, **183**, 183
family diagrams 4
Family Life Space Drawing (FLSD) 15–17; communication theory and 34–35; with couples (see couples, FLSD with); early research of 174–176; Experiences in Close Relationship Survey (ECR-R) and 188–196; expressive therapy techniques and 35; with families (see families, FLSD with); Family Assessment Measure (FAM-III) and 181–188; field theory and 31–34, 32; in foster care and termination of parental rights (see foster care and adoption, FLSD in); with individuals (see individual FLSD); insight through symbolic representation of 49; interpreting the symbolic representations of 51; introduction to 1–2; materials needed for 39–40; obtaining client information with 56–57; in psychiatric settings (see psychiatric settings, FLSD in); as research device 176–178; in school settings (see school settings, FLSD in); short-term multidimensional family intervention (STMFI) and 22–27, 36; step eight: communication lines 44–45; step five: environmental or institutional factors 42–43; step four: placement of significant people 41–42; step nine: reflecting with the family 45–46; step one: introducing the process 40; step seven: optional symbols-number one concern, greatest frustration 44; step six: identifying stress factors 44; step ten: developing the treatment plan 46; step three: family members each draw a personal symbol 40–41; step two: facilitator draws the first symbol 40; symbolic

interactionism and 36–37; symbolic interpretation in (*see* symbolic interpretation in FLSD); symbols used in (*see* symbols, FLSD); systems theory and 30–31; ten steps to complete 39–46; used with different types of clients 71–72; in various counseling settings 153–157
family mapping 7–8, 9, 14
family systems therapy 4
family therapy: cognitive behavioral 10–11; experiential model of 7–8; genogram process in 4–5, 5; models of 4; narrative 12, 12–13; psychodynamic 8–10; solution-focused 11, 11; strategic approach to 5–6; structural approach to 6–7, 6–7; systems theory and 3–4
feedback loops 34
Ferraro, F. 179
field theory 31–34, 32
FLSD *see* Family Life Space Drawing (FLSD)
foster care and adoption, FLSD in 154–155, 157; environmental symbols in 161, 165; placement of self in **158**, 158; placement of significant others in 159, 159–161, **160**, **164**, 164–165; stress symbols in 161
Fraley, R. C. 196
Freeman, A. 10
Fry, W., Jr. 34

Geddes, M. 39, 43, 46, 166, 175
Gennari, M. 35, 178, 196
genogram process 4–5, 5
Ghanbaripanah, A. 14
good communication line symbol 48
graphic visual techniques 7–8, 14
Grauf-Grounds, C. 153
greatest frustration symbol 48, 55–56, 68; in FLSD with couples 113

Haley, J. 5, 34
Hartman, A. 8
heterosexual couples, FLSD with 104–114
holistic dimension of STMFI 23

ideal family representations 57
ideal placements 58, 58–59
immigrants, FLSD with 156
individual FLSD: communication lines in 85–86, 93; environmental symbols in 76, 76–77, **77**, 82–83, **83**, 83, 89–91, **90**, 90; introduction to 73; placement of self and significant others in 74, 74–76, **75**, 80–82, **81**, 81, 86–89, 87, **88**; stress symbols in 77–79, 78, **84**, 84, 84–85, 91, 91–93, **92**; summary of 93–94
inner zone 52, 52–53
institutional symbols 47
interpretation, symbolic *see* symbolic interpretation in FLSD
interviewing 13

Jackson, D. 5, 34
Jung, C. 39

Kerr, M. 4
Knisely, J. S. 155
Kwiatkowska, H. a. 35

large family symbol 46
Lavee, Y. 154
Lewin, K. 29, 31–33, 180
life space 33
Locke Wallace Marital Adjustment scale 10
Lothamer, J. 179

Madigan, M. P. 175
Man and His Symbols 39
mandala symbol 39
McGoldrick, M. 5
Mead, G. H. 29, 36
Mead, M. 29
Medway, J. 39, 43, 46, 166, 175
middle zone 52, 53
Minuchin, S. 6
Mostwin, D. 20–22, 29, 37, 43, 44–45, 153, 175, 196; art therapy and 35; case study by 176; control circle developed by 51, 52; on distances and closeness 55; life space concept and 33; on the mandala symbol 39; on network of relationships expressed symbolically 46; outer zone developed by 53; on positive positioning 178; short-term multidimensional family intervention (STMFI) and 23–27
Mustaffa, M. S. 14

narrative family therapy 12, 12–13
National Catholic School of Social Service (NCSSS) 21

INDEX

Nichols, M. P. 4, 8–10, 12, 31, 172
number one concern symbol 48, 55–56, 68; in FLSD with couples 113

observational measures 13
Okoniewski, L. 177
Olson, D. 10–11
outcome rating scales (ORS) 13
outer zone 52, 53

Patterson, J. 14, 15, 49, 153
Piercy, F. P. 154, 179
pilot studies, FLSD 180–181; Experiences in Close Relationship Survey (ECR-R) 188–196; Family Assessment Measure (FAM-III) 181–188; summary of 196
poor communication line symbol 49
poverty, FLSD used in supporting people in 155–156
Preister, S. 24, 30
psychiatric settings, FLSD in 162; communication lines in 165–166; distance of symbols in 165; environmental and stress symbols in 165; placement of self in 163, 163–164, **164**; placement of significant others in **164**, 164–165
psychodynamic family therapy 8–10
purpose and value of family assessment 14

qualitative measures 13

Redmond, M. V. 36
research: early STMFI and FLSD 174–176; on expressive graphic techniques 179–180; Family Assessment Measure (FAM-III) 181–188; FLSD as tool for 176–178; future of FLSD 180, 196–197; other uses of FLSD in 179

same-sex couples, FLSD with 95–104
Satir, V. 7
school settings, FLSD in 167–168; communication lines in 169–170; environmental factors in 168; placement of family members in 168, 169; placement of significant others in 168, **168**; stress symbols in 169
self, placement of 60, **60**, 60; Experiences in Close Relationship Survey (ECR-R) and (*see* Experiences in Close Relationship Survey (ECR-R)); Family Assessment Measure (FAM-III) in couples (*see* Family Assessment Measure (FAM-III) and FLSD); in FLSD with couples 96, **97**, 97, 104, **105**, 105, 114–116, **115**, 115; in FLSD with families 126–128, **127**, 127, 141, 141–142, **142**; in foster care and termination of parental rights **158**, 158; in individual FLSD 74, 74–76, **75**, 80–82, **81**, 81, 86–89, 87, **88**; in psychiatric settings 163, 163–164, **164**
self-report measures 13
short-term multidimensional family intervention (STMFI) 22–27, 36, 179; early research of 174–176
significant others, placement of 61, 61–63, **62**; Experiences in Close Relationship Survey (ECR-R) and (*see* Experiences in Close Relationship Survey (ECR-R)); Family Assessment Measure (FAM-III) in couples (*see* Family Assessment Measure (FAM-III) and FLSD); in FLSD with couples 96–100, 98, **99**, 106–108, **107**, 107, 116, 116–119, **117**; in FLSD with families 128–131, **129**, **130**, 130, 142–145, 143, **144**; in foster care and termination of parental rights 159, 159–161, **160**, **164**, 164–165; in individual FLSD 74, 74–76, **75**, 80–82, **81**, 81, 86–89, 87, **88**; in psychiatric settings **164**, 164–165; in school settings 168, **168**
size of symbols 55
small symbol 47
social dimension of STMFI 23
social service settings, FLSD in 154
solution-focused family therapy 11, *11*
so-so communication line symbol 48
spatial dimension of STMFI 23
Sperry, L. 13
Stachowiak, J. 7
steps in completing the FLSD process 39–46
strategic approach to family counseling 5–6
stress symbols 47, 66, 66–67, **67**, 68; in FLSD with couples 101–103, **102**, 102, 111–113, **112**, 112, 121–124, 122, **123**; in FLSD with families 134–137, 135, **135–136**, 148–151, 149, **150**; in foster care and termination of parental rights 161, 165; in individual FLSD 77–79, 78, **84**, 84, 84–85, 91, 91–93, **92**; in psychiatric settings 165; in school settings 169
structural approach to family counseling 6–7, *6–7*

Sundet, R. 15
symbolic interaction dimension of STMFI 23
symbolic interactionism 36–37
symbolic interpretation in FLSD 51; case example 59, 68–70, 69; control circle and 51–52, 52; distances and closeness in 55; environmental symbols in **64**, 64, 64–66; ideal family representations and 57; ideal placements 58, 58–59; inner zone 52, 52–53; middle zone 52, 53; number one concern and greatest frustration symbols in 55–56, 68; obtaining client information with 56–57; other placements 53–54; outer zone 52, 53; placement of self and 60, **60**, 60; placement of significant others and 61, 61–63, **62**; placement of symbols and 54; size of symbols 55; stress symbols in 66, 66–67, **67**, **68**
symbols, FLSD 46–49; control circle 51–52, 52; distances and closeness of 55, 165; ideal placements of 58, 58–59; inner zone 52, 52–53; middle zone 52, 53; number one concern and greatest frustration 48, 55–56; other placements with 53–54; outer zone 52, 53; placement of 54; size of 55
systems theory 3–4, 30–31

Tafuri, S. 172
Tamanza, G. 35, 178
Taschman, A. 7
Teilhard de Chardin, P. 29
Thomlison, B. 13, 15, 172

unmarried couples with children, FLSD with 114–124

Wampold, B. 15, 16
Weakland, J. 34
Whelley, J. N. 26
Whitaker, C. 7
White, M. 12, 13
Williams, L. 14, 15, 49, 153
Wirsching, W. 179
World Health Organization 171

Yeakel, J. 179

PGMO 07/03/2019